T0131723

WHAT WILL MY BABY LOOK LIKE?

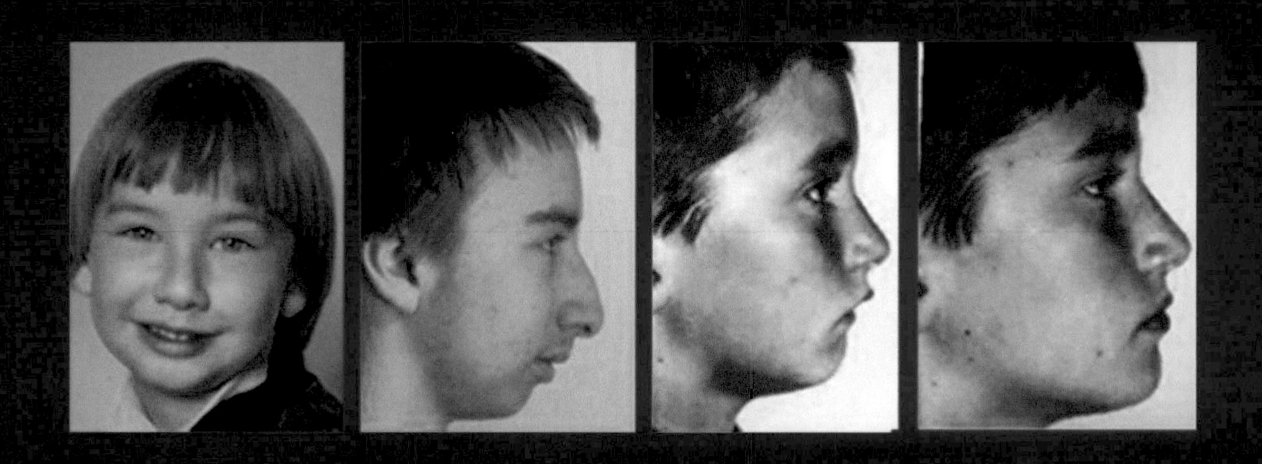

by

Professor John Mew

AuthorHouse™ UK
1663 Liberty Drive
Bloomington, IN 47403 USA
www.authorhouse.co.uk
UK TFN: 0800 0148641 (Toll Free inside the UK)
UK Local: 02036 956322 (+44 20 3695 6322 from outside the UK)

This book is printed on acid-free paper.

ISBN: 978-1-6655-9998-6 (sc)
ISBN: 978-1-6655-9997-9 (e)

Print information available on the last page.

Published by AuthorHouse 08/09/2022

authorHOUSE®

CONTENTS

CHAPTER 1

WHAT GOES WRONG

This short book explains why the position of a baby's tongue is largely responsible for their future appearance and why they should not be weened until their tongue posture is correct.

First, I need to explain how a baby's head and face develops. I will try to keep this simple but actually it is a very complex process. At conception the male sperm enters the female egg and gestation commences. To begin with the fertilized cell divides into two and then four and then eight cells. By then the cells 'know' which of them will form the head, the feet, and each side.

Amazingly each of these minute cells also 'knows' the shape of the entire body, and carries all the information which will determine the emotions and desires of the future child, even deciding when he or she will be ready to fall in love. Almost more surprisingly each cell 'knows' the exact shape of the ideal male or female face to the nearest millimetre or two.

We know this from the process of "cloning" where the nucleus of a female egg is replaced with a nucleus taken from the body of a male. The fertilized egg will grow into an identical twin of the male donor.

It used to be thought that growth was controlled by 'centres' in the body or electronic differentials, or hormones, or by neighbouring cells, but in 1985 I put forward the Cell Volition Theory (CVT). About 3 billion years ago in evolutionary history, individual cells started to group together to form multicellular animals and this required cooperation, organisation and perhaps leadership.

The Cell Volition Theory suggests that each cell has a map of the whole body and does its best to obey that. Although they work and even die for the benefit of their host, they still maintain some self-will (volition). Of the many competing theories I believe this to be the most logical.

Anyway, each cell divides millions of times, forming the different parts of the body and this process appears to be guided by sheaths of fascia which surround teach area enabling them to grow individually until they are ready to join together to create major sections of the body. Most of this is complete by the twelfth week of gestation.

The face grows as three projections from behind. The upper jaw (the Maxilla) grows as two halves, while the lower jaw (the Mandible) develops separately underneath it, each within their fascial sheath and these processes then join up to form the face, almost at the end of gestation. At the point where the cells surrounding each sheath meet, some need to die so that the various processes are able to fuse together. This process of cell death is called apoptosis and is a major feature during our growth. In fact it continues throughout life, so that almost our whole body is replaced every ten years or so. Sometimes apoptosis fails and the sheaths are unable to join together resulting in cleft lips, palates or Spina Bifida.

The Tongue.

The tongue develops as a small bulge in the floor of the mouth, before growing into a powerful muscular organ. Primarily it acts as a three-way valve, to seal off the mouth, the nose or the throat (trachea) but it also performs many other duties, placing food between the teeth, scouring for loose particles and of course speech. Perhaps most vitally, it acts in conjunction with the mandible to express the milk from the breast. This is what we need to talk about.

The developed tongue is attached by ligaments to the various bones around it, mainly to the hyoid, below it, but also to the mandible beside it and the skull, above it. Muscles can only lengthen or shorten in straight lines, so to move the tongue in various directions, different muscles have to lengthen or contract.

Tongue Ties. Changes in shape of the body of the tongue are achieved by the intrinsic muscles. These are placed in different planes, and are attached partially to each other and partially to the fascial sheaths which run between them. This gives some people enough anchorage to extend the tongue tip to their nose or chin. However the fascia of a few people remains tight and restricts tongue movement.

During breast feeding the tongue pushes firmly on the breast but when infants are bottle or spoon fed, the tongue is much less active. As a result the natural apoptosis of the facia may not take place, and some of the 'Fascial Ties' remain, these may subsequently need to be stretched or cut. We will discuss this in more detail later.

Swallowing. The dictionary definition of swallowing is "To cause food, drink, pills etc to move from your mouth into your stomach". While this may be an oversimplification, most mammals swallow in a similar manner starting with the tongue pushing up on to the palate before the centre is dropped to initiate a peristaltic wave which carries the bolus down the throat (oesophagus). Interestingly most civilised humans do not swallow like that. They suck on their teeth collapsing the dentition and frequently creating narrow palates and receding jaws; why is this?

Posture. Many years ago, I realized that most deformed jaws were due to oral para-function and especially posture. This has been difficult to confirm, as long-term posture is almost impossible to measure. After some research I suggested (Mew 1981) that "the tongue should rest on the palate with the lips sealed and the teeth in or near contact". I also suggested that if this posture was maintained, the face and dentition would grow as nature intended. I called this theory the Tropic Premise, because the pattern of facial growth was in some ways similar to the way plants respond to sunlight and gravity.

My theory was broadly rejected by professionals at the time but 40 years later it has become popular with the public who call it 'mewing' and I am told that some 50,000,000 youngsters and adults around the world currently practice it. There can be no doubt that oral posture has some influence on Dento-Facial development even if we are not quite sure how it works.

The Tropic Premise describes how poor posture can damage the development of the human face but it did not explain the reason why oral posture goes wrong in the first place. I put forward the Mastantlos Hypothesis (Mew 2020) to provide a logical explanation for the initial cause as well.

Because oral posture cannot be measured both these theories remain without proof, but like the apple which fell on Newton's head, many of the leaps in science have come from observational Hypotheses.

Life-Style. In my opinion poor facial growth is due to three things –

1/ **Living Indoors** where there are high levels of household dust. Much of this is allergenic and causes irritation to the mucous membrane lining the nose. This may cause it to swell, partially blocking the nasal airway, which naturally encourages mouth breathing. If this happens more than a few times a child is likely to develop an 'open mouth' habit. Long-term mouth breathing is known to disrupt growth causing a narrow down growing face, especially if it occurs between the ages of six and twenty. (see picture 1)

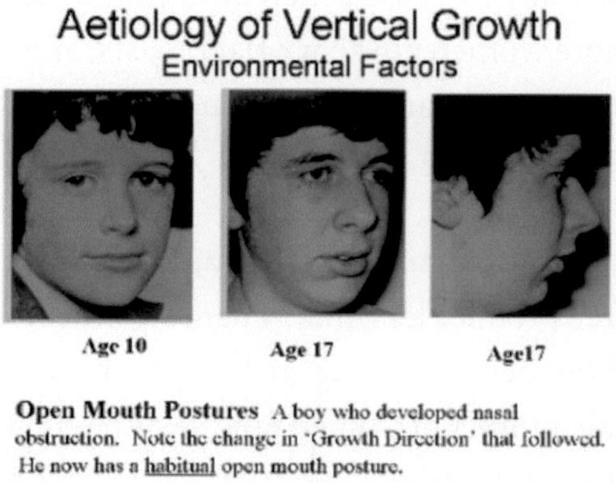

Aetiology of Vertical Growth
Environmental Factors

Age 10 | Age 17 | Age17

Open Mouth Postures A boy who developed nasal obstruction. Note the change in 'Growth Direction' that followed. He now has a habitual open mouth posture.

Picture 1

2/ **Soft Food.** Most animals chew with strong jaw muscles and sometimes they may die for no other reason than they have worn their teeth away. Our own ancestors used to wear their teeth down almost to the gum by the time they were 60. Nowadays our food is so soft that many people show little sign of wear at any age. This is one of the main reasons that our muscles are much weaker now and why our faces tend to lengthen.

3/ **Shortened Breastfeeding.** No one knows exactly how long our ancestors breast fed for but most mammals continue breastfeeding until after the 'milk' teeth arrive. In Humans this is about 24 months. However, many parents start weening soon after birth. No other mammals do this and yet I hear some professionals encouraging young mothers to provide water and liquified food to infants using spoons, cups, or bottles. This is certainly unnatural and in my experience is likely to disrupt tongue posture.

Weening Matters. Currently the average period of human suckling appears to be about six months although there are areas and groups where breastfeeding is longer or shorter. You often see mothers spoon feeding their child and having to collect residue from around their lips and re-insert it. They are teaching them to swallow unnaturally so they are likely to grow up with flat cheeks, big noses and receding jaws.

Primitive mothers had no means of providing liquid supplements, but after about one year used to chew lumps of meat and vegetable before giving them to their child. Gill Rapley author of 'baby led weening' (Rapley 2019) suggests that babies should be allowed to decide when they wish to start chewing their food.

Milk Supply. In our modern world many mothers have difficulty providing enough milk and so switch to spoon, cup or bottle. As I have said I am sure this disrupts the child's future growth and appearance, but what is the alternative? Interestingly, this problem rarely occurred in primitive societies.

As society developed the wealthy began to employ wet nurses and in Ancient Greece, they were accepted as members of high society. By 1600, it is suggested that over half of European women were sending their babies to be nursed by other women. However, in 1794, the Germans reversed this making it a legal requirement that all healthy women breastfed their babes. So you can see the history of breast feeding has swung like a pendulum, controlled, some say, by men who consider the more a woman lactates the fewer babies she has.

Over the last two hundred years, the increasing use of contraceptives has encouraged women to take a greater role in the workplace. This has naturally increased their ambition which in turn has altered their hormone distribution. Possibly as a result more women now have flat breasts, and narrow hips. Also in nature women mated soon after puberty but due to rising standards of education, new laws prevent intercourse under the age of 15 to 18 depending on where you live.

We do not know what difference this makes to rearing infants but older mothers are likely to have greater difficulties with conception and often produce less milk. There are other factors too. Children who are brought up with the idea that early sexual intercourse is wrong are likely to menstruate later and their anatomy may be affected permanently. An increasing number of women now delay having children until they have established themselves in business, often waiting until 40 or over. All these factors may restrict initial milk flow.

Anyone who has seen a new baby crawl across their mothers stomach to their breast and 'latch on' will know how important this process is. Many maternity units do not encourage it and that may also be a reason why a number of babies fail to 'latch on'.

Lactation is a complex process and if a lamb dies, its mother may not let another lamb suckle, unless it is first covered by the skin of its own dead offspring. Also if a sheep is anaesthetised before a birth, so they feel no pain, they will frequently reject their offspring. When you consider that all these processes are totally instinctive it is hardly surprising that things sometimes go wrong.

One of the greatest problems is when the baby fails to 'latch on'. As we have been discussing this seems more common in highly civilised countries and possibly with older, more ambitious mothers. It is usually a sign of lack of milk but sometimes the baby only seems to want to suck the nipple. In such cases the 'Flipple' technique may be helpful. This involves pushing as much of the mothers breast into the babies mouth as possible and encouraging babies to pump the breast as suggested in the Mastantlos Hypothesis.

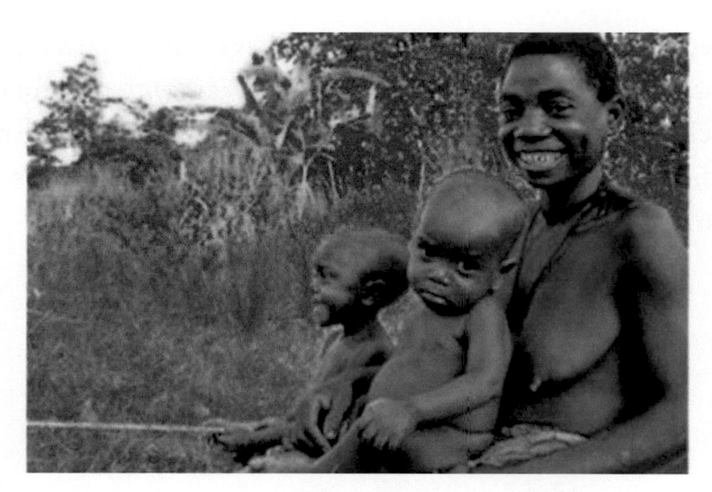

Picture 2

This influences the natural shape of the breast. I personally think this is important, for the development of a wide forward growing face and ultimately a good looking child. (see picture 2)

If the baby does not 'latch on' and fails to suckle satisfactorily then obviously they need to be fed by other means, but I have no doubt that this is not natural and that spoon, cup or bottle feeding will result in facial deformation. However I believe that one day human ingenuity will create a plastic breast that allows a baby to suckle with a pump action.

Pacifiers. It has been suggested that "75-85% of all children in western countries use pacifiers" and that "Children weaned from breastfeeding early, use a pacifier more often than those who are breastfed longer". This should not surprise us as monkeys will often suck their thumbs if separated from their mothers too early. Nearly all pacifiers disrupt natural tongue posture and inevitably there is a long-term price to pay for this.

Natural Breast Feeding..

Recent research (Elad 2014) suggests that "Breast-feeding is the outcome of a dynamic synchronization between oscillation of the infant's mandible, rhythmic motility of the tongue, and the Breast Milk Ejection Reflex (MER) that drives maternal milk toward the nipple outlet".

I am sure that this is an accurate description of the rhythmic movement of the mandible and tongue against the breast, but I am not so certain about the "milk ejection reflex", because the only muscles in the breast, help to erect the nipple. There is a lattice of myoepithelial cells that surround the alveoli, but it was established many years ago (Ellendorff 1982) that the milk pressure in the mammalian breasts is around 0.045 Bar (1.26 PSI). This seems insufficient to eject the milk down collapsible ducts in the quantities required, without some assistance.

I believe that additional force is required from the action of the tongue supported by the mandible, which pushes on a mouthful of breast to assist in extracting the milk which is then swallowed by a peristaltic wave starting in the middle of the tongue.

Sucking is not a very effective way of moving fluids as it relies on atmospheric pressure and unsupported ducts are likely to collapse, unless held open by cartilage, as they are with the bronchi of the lungs. Pumping is far more effective and clearly can be related to the rhythmic movements of the mandible and the tongue, as observed by Elad. Additional support for this concept comes from my own research on the palatal rugae (Mew 1974). (see picture 3)

Tongue Posture

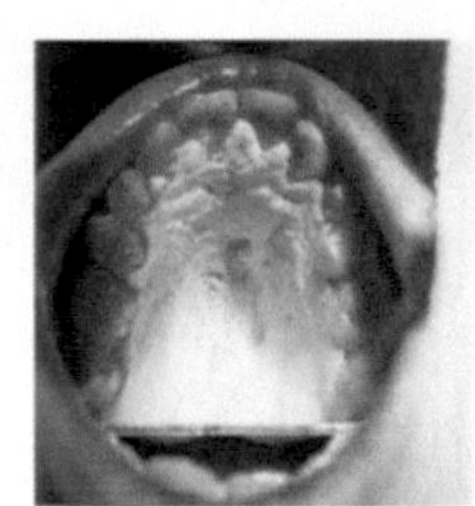

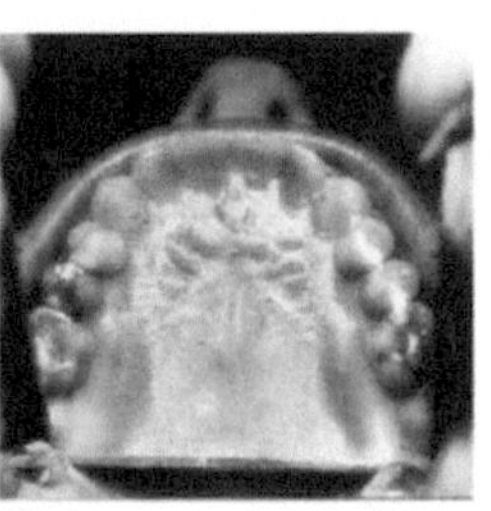

The palates of both these patients were painted with indicator paste and they were asked to swallow three times. The difference in the area of contact between the broad and narrow palate is obvious.

Picture 3

This showed that narrow Palates are associated with lack of tongue contact, while wide palates go with broad contact from the tongue and flattened palatal rugae.

Watch this video on Facebook 19.3.22 to see how the tongue should stay 'glued' to the palate https://www.facebook.com/groups/craniofacialactiongroup/posts/4950911344985176/ . If the tongue does not do this then the whole maxilla will be narrow, sometimes exceedingly so. I believe that the width between the upper first molars should be around 44 millimetres for an adult male and 42 for a woman. However the average in the United Kingdom is around 33½. This is why so many people have flat cheeks big noses and reseeding chins which in my opinion is primarily due to lack of full-term breast feeding.

At about six months the front teeth start to erupt. We tend to think of the teeth and bone being rigid but actually they are moved and shaped by very light forces. Again my research suggest 1 or 2 grams (the force from a feather) will guide an erupting tooth into position and the jaw bone will then hold it there firmly. This is why tongue position is so important.

If the tongue rests against the palate as it should do, the upper teeth will erupt around it in a broad curve. If at the same time the lips are sealed then they will do so in a regular line. It is really very simple, but only about 5% of humans keep their tongue on their palate, which seems a similar ratio of those who are breast fed to full term without premature weening.

Tongue Ties. Many babies and young children are born with tongue ties. That is because the fascial fibres which should apoptize at birth fail to do so. In my experience they usually free themselves following vigorous breastfeeding, but if they fail to do so they may need cutting or stretching. The incidence of tongue ties has increased recently, this may be due to increased diagnosis, or reduced breastfeeding but residual ties do seem related to tongue function and if this is not rectified, the ties often reattach after they are cut.

The Indicator Line This is the distance between the tip of the nose and the edge of the upper front teeth. It is an important measurement because it tells you the approximate position of the upper jaw. For a child of four it should be about 27 millimetres and increase about 1 millimetre a year until puberty.

Some people think it just measures the size of the nose but actually the nasal bones are firmly attached to the forehead. If a child leaves their mouth open, the middle section of their face including their maxilla and the teeth will drop (grow) down leaving the nose behind. As a result the nose appears to stick out from the flattened cheeks, although actually it has hardly moved. (see pictures 4, 5 and 6)

Measuring the Indicator Line will tell you how your child will look and where the maxilla is now to the nearest few millimetres. The higher the Indicator Line the longer the face will be. See pictures

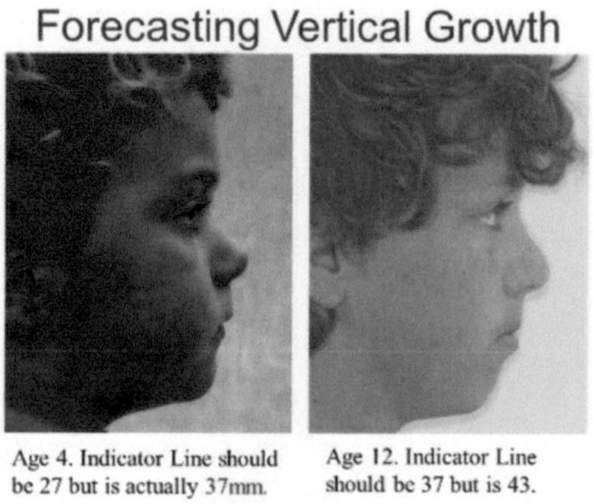

Forecasting Vertical Growth

Age 4. Indicator Line should be 27 but is actually 37mm.

Age 12. Indicator Line should be 37 but is 43.

Picture 4

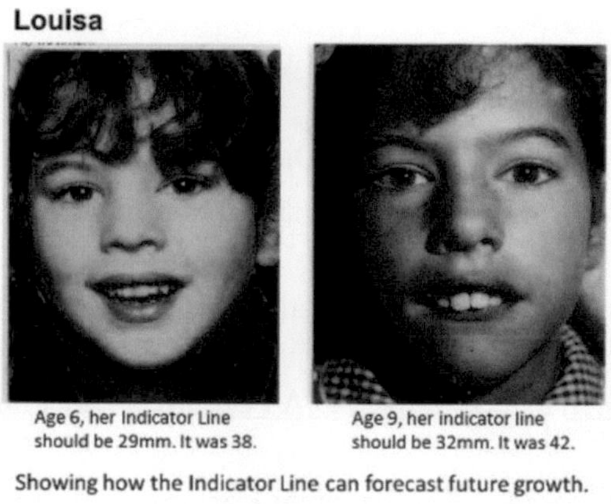

Louisa

Age 6, her Indicator Line should be 29mm. It was 38.

Age 9, her indicator line should be 32mm. It was 42.

Showing how the Indicator Line can forecast future growth.

Picture 5

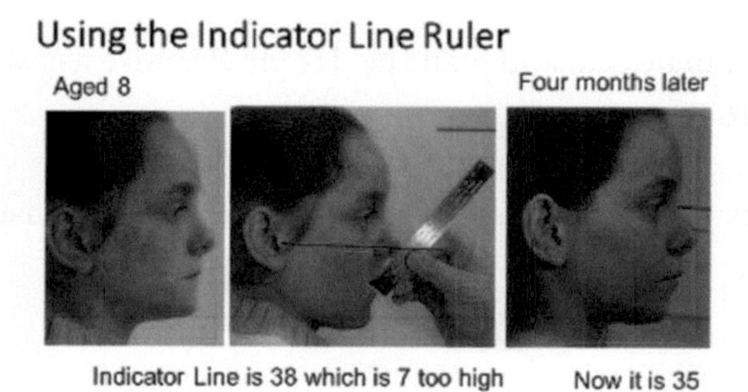

Picture 6

There is also a **Lower Indicator Line** which recommends the correct position of the lower incisors relative to the mandible. If it is too high the incisors will be too far back and the chin will look pointed (see pictures 7 and 8). Idealy it should be two millimetres less than the Upper Indicator Line at the same age.

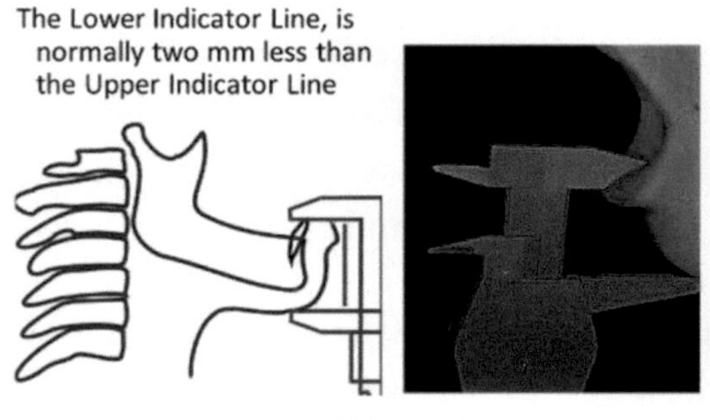

Picture 7

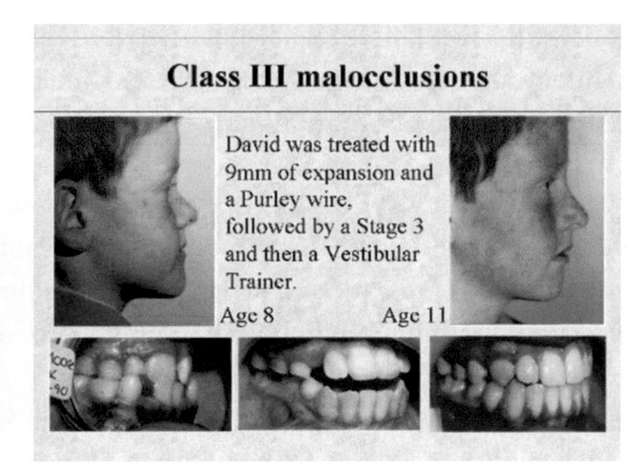

Picture 8

References.

Elad D, Kozlovsky P, Blum O, Laine A F, Po M J, Botzer E, Dollberg S, Zelicovich M, and Sira L B. 2014 Biomechanics of Milk Extraction During Breast Feeding. Proc Natl Acad Sci. 2014;111: 5230–5235.

Facebook Video. "Craniofacial Action Group" 19.3.22

F Ellendorff, M L Forsling, D A Poulain. 1982 The milk ejection reflex in the pig. J Physiol 1982;333:577-94.

Mew, JRC 1974. "The Incisive Foramen - A Possible Reference Point". British Journal of Orthodontics. 1:4. 143-146 1974

Mew,J.R.C. "The aetiology of malocclusion: can the Tropic Premise assist our understanding". British Dental Journal. 1981:**151;** :296-302.

Mew. JRC. Mastantlos Kasetsu, - Hitonoennge, Zetsuno posuchaa, Zetsushoutai Tanshukushou. . Jap J Ortho Pract . 2020; 57-65".

Rapley G and Murkett T. Baby-led Weaning: Helping your baby to love good food (2nd Edn). 2019. Vermilion, London.

CHAPTER 2

HOW BREAST FEEDING AFFECTS THE FACE

How Breastfeeding Affects the Face. Few undamaged skulls have survived from our Palaeolithic past but their first molars appeared to be nearly 50 millimetres apart. I am told that Brazilian mothers used to suspend their babies in the air with their thumb against their palate to ensure good forward growth. Currently the average inter-molar width varies from country to country and the 33½mm average in the United Kingdom (Mew 2012) leaves insufficient room to accommodate a full dentition of 32 teeth.

Most mammals suckle their young until the first permanent molars erupt, while primitive human mothers probably breast fed until 2.8 years (Bogin 2007). As I said earlier when the baby was ready, mothers used to feed them soft or pre-chewed food, (baby led weaning). This probably began soon after the Incisors erupted at around 10 months and increased as the baby molars started to erupt at about 18 months.

The ratio of particulate food continued to increase as the last of the 'milk' teeth erupted at around 24 months, by when they could chew quite tough food. However breast milk still formed a significant part of their diet until final termination of breastfeeding around 30 months. Remember that before cups and spoons, only the breast could provide an infant with water.

For several centuries now humans have progressively supplemented breastfeeding with bottle feeding and strong views are expressed about the rival merits of each. It is not my intention to make recommendations but to consider the mechanics of breastfeeding and its possible long-term consequences on tongue posture, and facial development, hoping this will assist you to make your own decisions.

Oral Posture. Long-term oral posture is very difficult to measure accurately and this has discouraged researchers who like to be precise, As a result the influence of oral posture on the face and dentition has been largely ignored and few recommendations have been made for mothers. When evidence is absent, a logical hypothesis may be all we have.

The philosopher Karl Popper taught, "it is not possible to prove anything, even if the sun will rise tomorrow" and suggested that it was more fruitful to examine all the hypotheses and adopt the one that fitted the evidence best. He lived near me as a youngster and strongly influenced my thinking. Accordingly, I have put forward two theories the 'Tropic Premise' and the 'Mastantlos Hypothesis' to explain how the teeth and surrounding bone should develop. Viewed conversely, the same theories help us to understand why so many people have narrow maxillae and retruded mandibles.

Recognising Poor Oral Posture.

With experience, a clinician can recognise the effect of poor posture on the appearance of both children and adults. What do they look for? It might be best to start with correct posture and development. If, as the Tropic Premise suggests, the tongue rests on the palate from birth with the lips sealed and the teeth are in or near contact, then the face and teeth will be near ideal. I show the face of Dolly Alderton the Sunday Times columnist. (see picture 9)

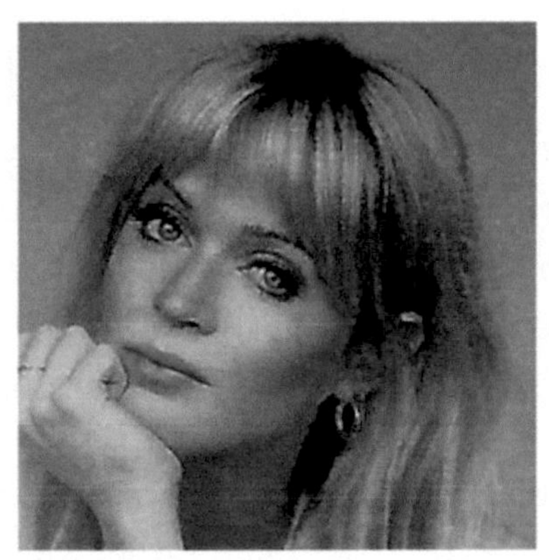

Dolly Alderton curtesy of Sunday Times..

Picture 9

The features to look at are her upright forehead, her forward placed cheek bones, her relatively small nose, the broad upper and lower jaws, with a suggestion of dimples on each side. The shape of her lips are appealing although her lower is slightly large, possibly because her hand is resting on her chin. Each of these features is due to specific aspects of her oral posture.

Even at the age of 8 changing your mouth posture can make a significant change to the shape of your face and position of your teeth. The boy in this picture could not afford treatment but with training, was able to change his own mouth posture and you can see the major changes in his face in just one year. It widened considerably with no active treatment but of real significance, his severely rotated canine tooth aligned spontaneously. (see picture 10)

Oral Myotherapy

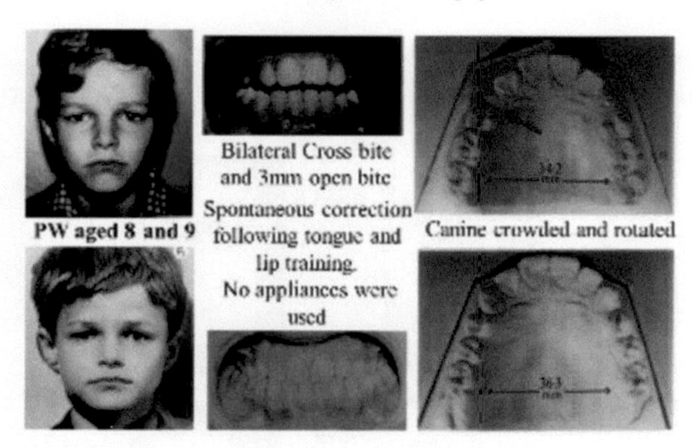

Picture 10

Blocked Noses. If someone's airway becomes restricted, they tend to tilt their head back to make it easier to breathe. However, if this continues for long, their forehead will permanently slope back and their whole neck will tilt forward to balance the spine and in the tong-term the bones of your face and lower jaw willchange shape radically (See Pictures of a 10 year old girl who started to keep her mouth open). At the same time her whole spine re-adjusted. (see pictures 11 and 12)

Sometimes adverse muscle forces will disrupt normal growth

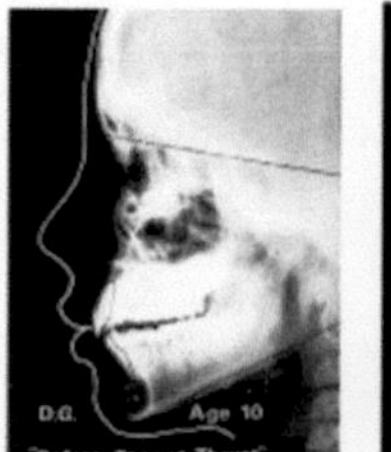

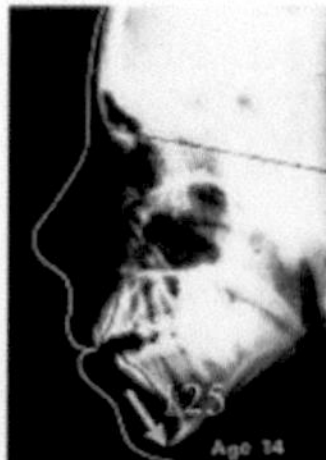

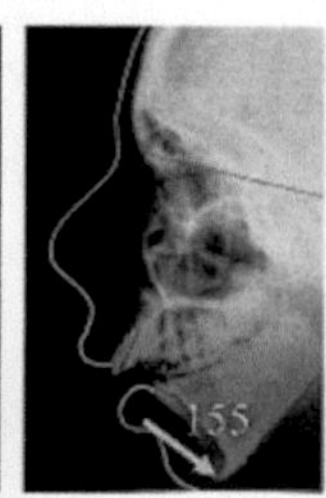

Parafunction. The effect of a lack of lip seal and a tongue between tooth posture (Mew 1981). The final face looks convex despite the fall back of the maxilla

Picture 11

Aetiology of Vertical Growth

How can we explain this?

The mandible of the previous girl aged 10 and 14.

Superimposed on inner cortical structures after Bjork. Note the horizontal ramus has shortened by one third during a period of maximum growth

Picture 12

As I said earlier, blocked noses are usually caused by allergies and the consequences of mouth breathing are severe. Allergens are most common in bedrooms because of dust from mites, clothes and bed covers. This dust can often be seen if a shaft of sunlight crosses the room. However, many new-born children are placed in bedrooms where they are likely to develop allergies and stuffy noses, so mouth breathing can easily become a habit.

I would recommend filtering the air in all bedrooms or alternatively laying the dust with an Ioniser. Blocked noses can be cleared by putting decongestants up a child's nose just before bedtime, but the nose is likely to block again if the lips separate, so I suggest putting tape across the lips until they run short of breath. You can try this for a little longer each night, until the child can sleep all night with the lips sealed, I still use tape myself.

Almost all children can achieve this, so don't give up. You might find it helpful to learn about Buteyko breathing.

Leaving your lips apert will also change the shape of the whole face. (see picture 13)

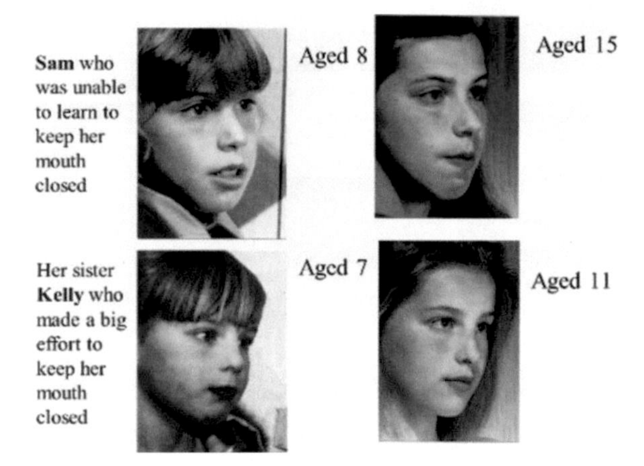

Picture 13

If you did not breast feed correctly, you probably suck when you swallow with your tongue touching your side teeth. Over 90% of bottle or spoon-fed children do this. If you try swallowing slowly you may feel your tongue suck on your teeth. This is what causes a narrow upper jaw (35 millimetres or less between your upper first molars). There may also be scalloping marks on the side of your tongue and your front teeth will probably overlap too much and the lower front teeth will be crowded. This type of swallow also causes your cheeks to look puffy and unattractive, whereas learning to swallow correctly will improve their shape and dimples will appear. (see picture 14 of 28 year old woman)

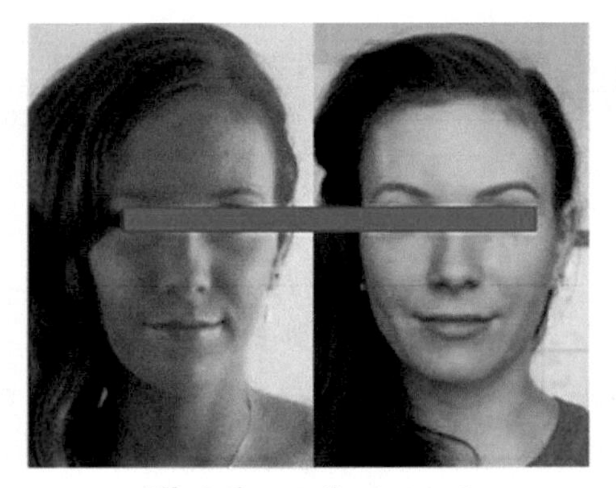

Affect of correcting tongue to cheek swallow between 28 and 30.

Picture 14

Open Bites. Many people touch their front teeth with their tongue when at rest, and as infants probably sucked a bottle or their thumb. As a result their tongue touches their front teeth and this is enough to prevent them meeting (an open bite, see picture 15). Treatment to improve the posture will correct that, first enlarge the upper jaw (see below) to make room for the tongue then train it to rest on the palate. If the tongue is in the right position, with the mouth kept closed the open bite will close and the face will be attractive. (see picture 15)

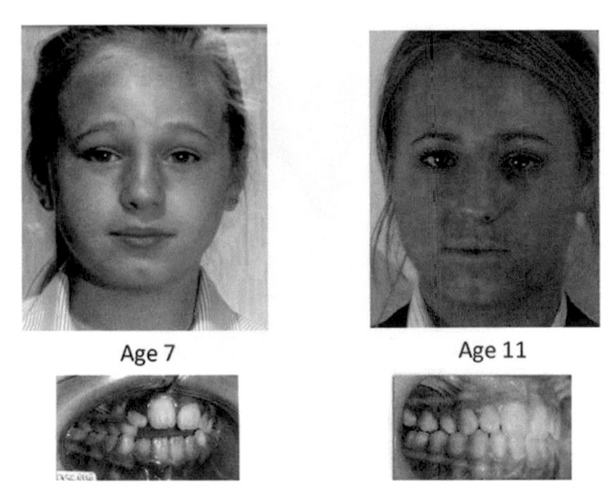

Picture 15

Widening the Jaws. If your tongue posture is wrong your upper jaw is likely to be narrow, however it is possible to widen it artificially; this is known as maxillary expansion. In youngsters it can be widened 15 millimetres or more with little tilting of the teeth. (see picture 16)

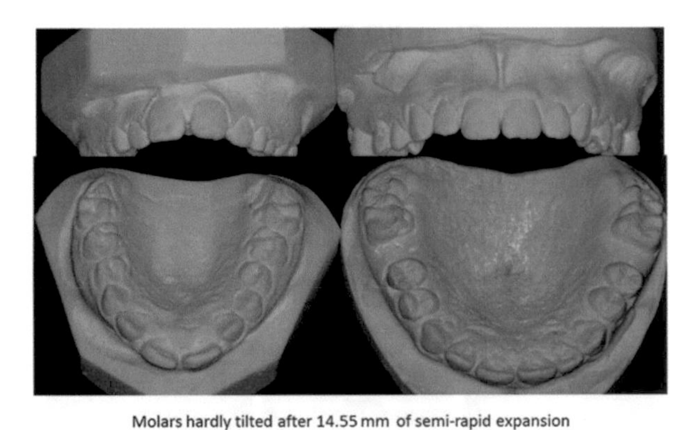

Molars hardly tilted after 14.55 mm of semi-rapid expansion

Improved shape of palate after removable orthotropic expansion.

Picture 16

This improves the appearance of the cheek bones in both young and old. (see pictures 17 and 18)

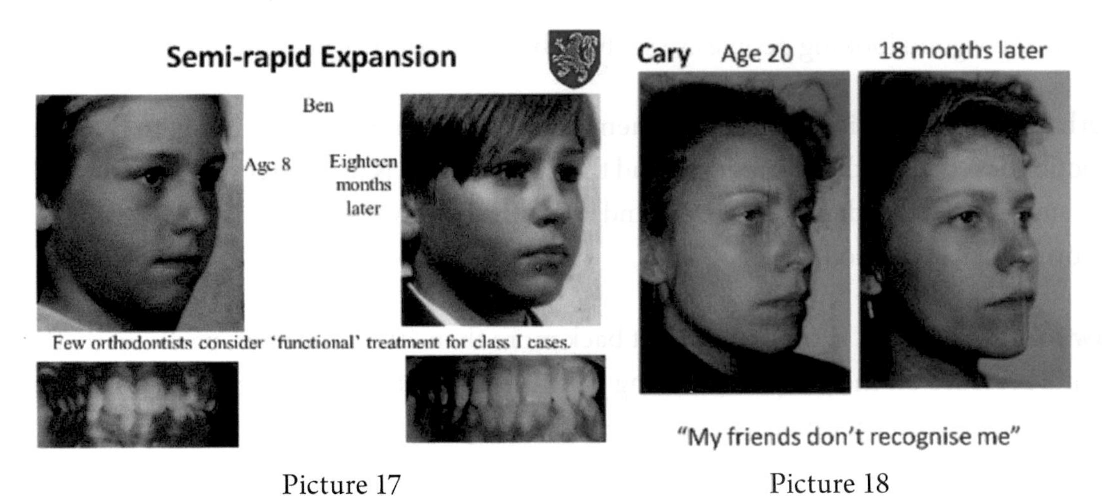

Picture 17

Picture 18

Some people worry that the lower jaw (mandible) will not fit the widened upper jaw but the width of both jaws is maintained by the tongue. If there is no tongue the jaw will be very narrow. (see picture 19)

Forecasting Vertical Growth

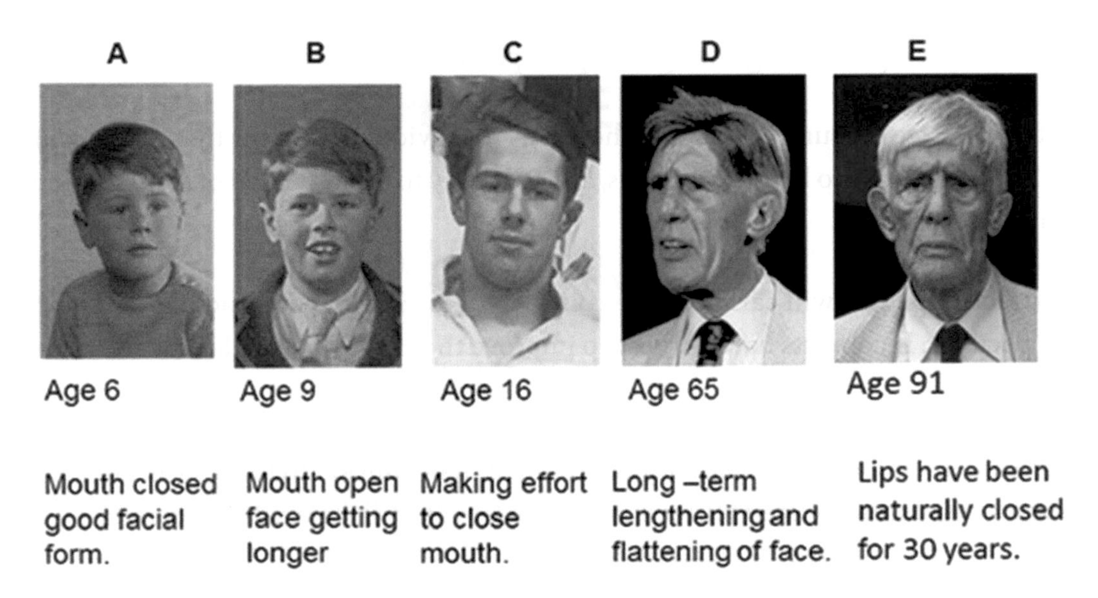

Picture 21

Sealed lips are so important that I tell mothers of young children to tap them on the head with a stick every time their lips are apart. It may be wearisome for both mother and child but it drives home the message, and over time is often successful.

The 'Orbicularis' muscle seals the lips, acting like a purse string, but some children close their mouths using the 'Mentalis' instead (the muscle underneath the lips) which lifts up the centre of the lower lip. You can see when they do this as their chin will often pucker and in the long-term the corners of the lip will drop giving them a glum look. Amazingly this can actually cause people to become glum because others read this into their personality. Also too much use of the Mentalis muscle tends to damage the gum in front of your lower front teeth and can even lead to their early loss. In addition, constant contraction of the mentalis will give you a sloping chin.

As I said at the beginning of this chapter the Tropic Premise should be the natural posture for all humans but in fact fewer than 10% posture and swallow like that.

We mentioned that most mammals swallow with their mouth closed but due to living indoors, eating soft food and shortened breastfeeding, the majority of humans let their jaws and tongues drop. This disrupts natural growth, causing narrow jaws, receding chins, big noses and flattened cheeks. Mewing does no more than promote your natural swallow and oral posture but the effect can be amazing.

Most adverse growth can be prevented if posture is corrected before the age of seven and be improved at almost any age by posturing and swallowing correctly, that is what mewing is. However, people who have swallowed incorrectly for many years find this difficult. The main problem is positioning the tongue, however the correct reflexes are still dormant in the mind and can be recovered if you make sufficient effort.

Your teeth are subject to the Tooth Eruption Mechanism (TEM) so they erupt when out of contact and intrude when in contact. Your face is longer when you wake up in the morning and shorter after a meal. This has evolved so that all the teeth meet evenly. Sadly because many people leave their mouths open too much, the TEM cannot work and their teeth meet unevenly. This often results in bruxing, clicking jaw joints and pain.

Swallowing. My instructions are simple; say "TING" and your tongue will be in the right position. It should rest there hardly touching the teeth unless you are talking or eating. At the same time your lips should be lightly sealed and your teeth either touching or nearly touching. Over the whole day they should be in contact for between four and eight hours so the TEM can work. The time varies depending on the force of contact.

We discussed the Mastantlos Hypothesis earlier which explains how children who are brought up with spoons and bottles tend have poor tongue posture and suck when they swallow when they should push. This is what causes narrow palates and if you swallow now, most of you will suck on your teeth rather than push on your palate. Changing that could make a big improvement to your life at any age.

I find patients often have considerable difficulty changing from a lifetime of sucking to pushing. It may help you if I describe some of the signs of a poor swallow. Firstly 'Scalloping' (marks on the side of the tongue) is a certain sign that you contact your teeth with your tongue. Scalloping is usually accompanied by a 'deep bite' (your front teeth overlap too much vertically) and often some of the teeth on one or even both sides of your mouth do not interdigitate correctly. This is hard to change but remember to push on your palate, not suck when you swallow.

Sometimes the front teeth don't touch unless the jaw is moved forward, this is because the tongue is touching them, remember a feather can move teeth if it is left there long enough. The tip of your tongue should rest on the rugae (the ridges in the gum behind your front teeth) not quite touching the teeth.

When people suck on their teeth to swallow, they need to contract their cheeks (Buccinator muscles) and lips to prevent air passing between the teeth. The contraction of these muscles can be seen by a slight contraction every time they swallow. With a correct swallow there should be no contraction of either the cheeks or lips, or indeed any other facial muscles, although your jaw muscles (the masseters) do contract slightly when your tongue pushes on your palate, you can feel this by resting your fingers on them each side.

My son Mike calls this the Mona Lisa swallow. You can test for this by asking them to swallow with their lips apart, He calls this a "cheesy" swallow. People who suck when they swallow find this difficult because they are used to contracting their cheek and lips or biting on their tongue to prevent air coming in between their teeth. Changing this habit can make a big difference to your appearance (See Illustration of 28 year old woman in chapter 2).

Lip Seal. Keeping the mouth closed is essential for attractive growth, I think more so than tongue posture. I feel so sad when I see children with their mouths wide open and feel tempted to tell all mothers of the damage it can do to their future appearance. On one occasion in a café, I warned the mother of a three year old who had his mouth wide open. Because I thought it would be unkind to say his face would be unattractive, I just said his teeth would be crooked.

Quite amazingly, I was in my clinic 14 years later when she recognized me and said I had been wrong and his teeth were quite straight. I was surprised and asked if I could see him. She agreed and arranged for him to come to the clinic. She was correct his teeth were fairly straight but his face was not so good! (see picture 22)

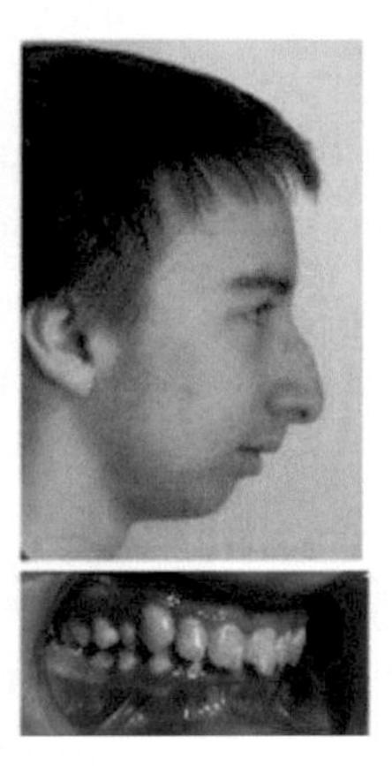

Picture 22

Many people send me pictures of the changes to their face after mewing. Sadly, few have taken good pictures of themselves before they started mewing, so the photographs are often hard to match. It is also possible to 'photo shop' faces so they look better (or worse), but there would be little reason for them to do that, when sending photos to me. I show some of them below and although several may be distorted, there can be no doubt that many have improved. (see pictures 23 to 33)

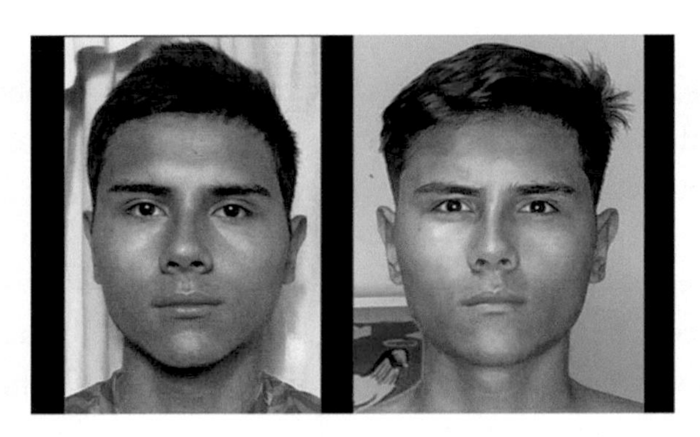

Fernando Cortez Avila four months mewing. Facebook 23.2.2021.

Picture 23

Put up by Kewickz on Reddit 'Orthotropics' Result of 2 years mewing from 17 to 19

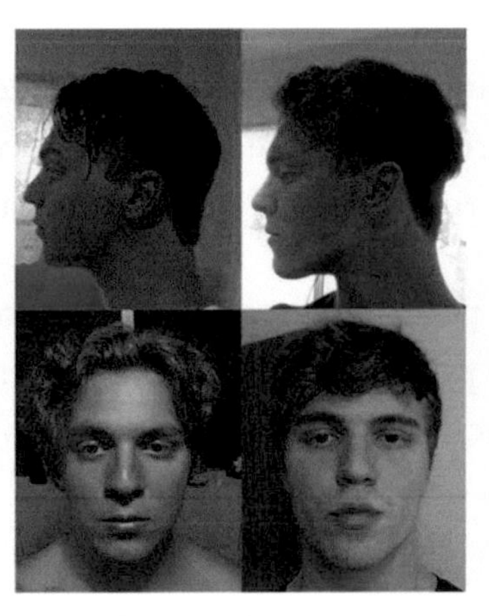

Picture 24

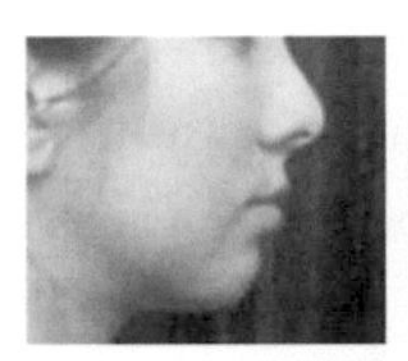

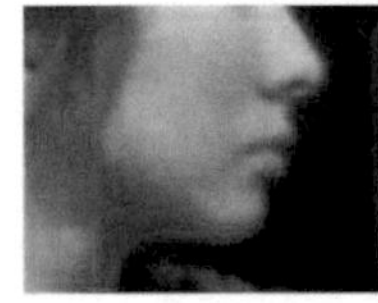

A 28 year old patient sent me these pictures after 'mewing' for 18 months.

Picture 25

Mewing for a period Facebook.

Picture 26

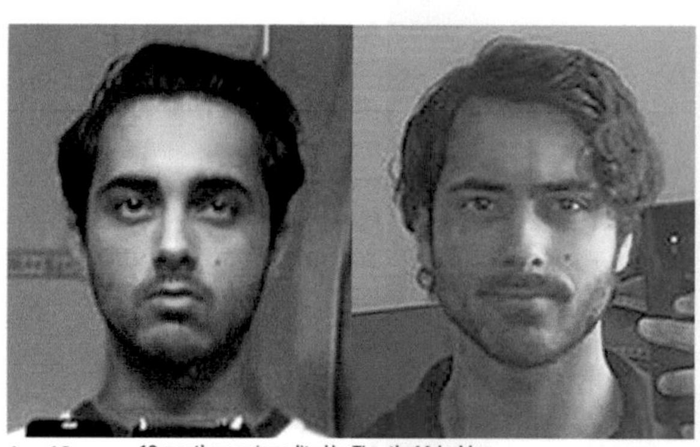

Age 18 18 months mewing edited by Timothy Mclochlan. Age 23

Picture 27

Age 16 from Reddit Age 21

The result of five years mewing. Note how the tongue to palate posture and swallow has caused the cheeks to flatten. Also the lip shape has improved because of improved lip seal

Picture 28

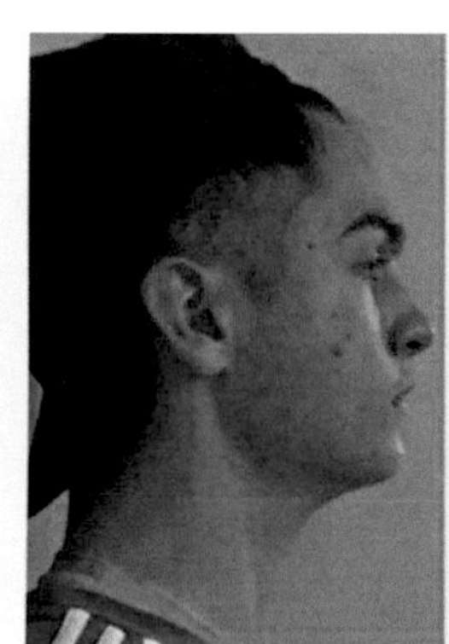

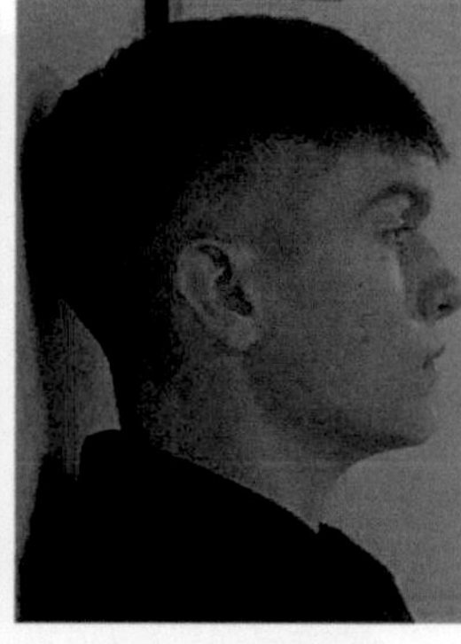

Nov. 2019 Mewing Nov. 2020

Picture 29

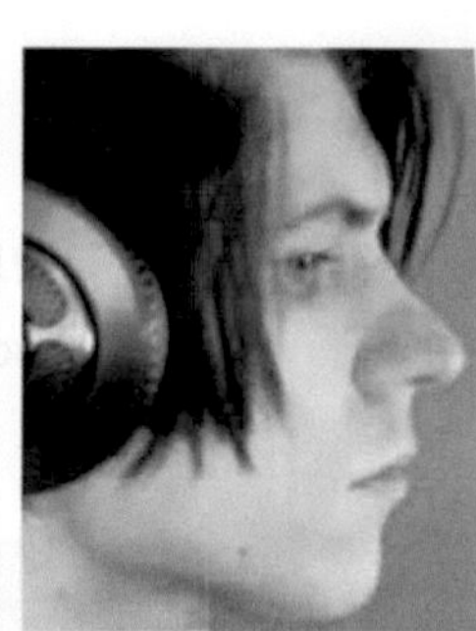

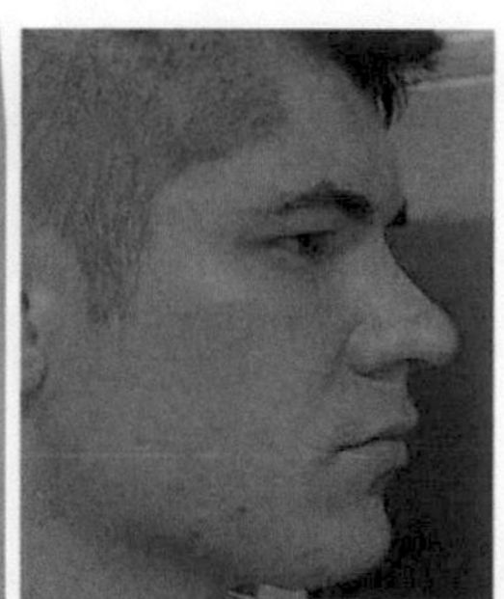

Age 20 Age 27, Mewing

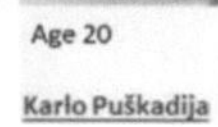

Karlo Puškadija

Picture 30

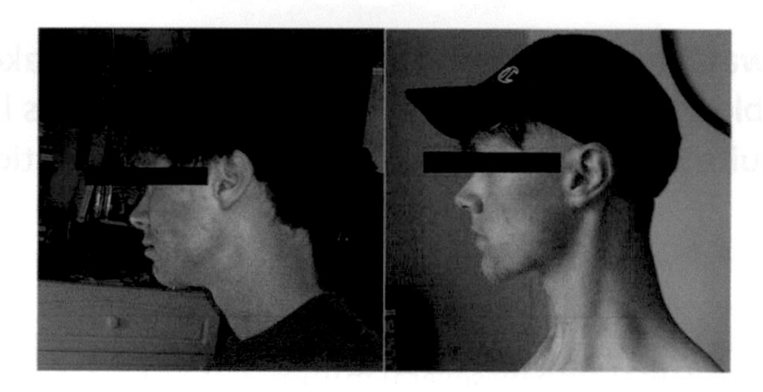

Eighteen months mewing from 2019 to 2000.. Weighed ~57kg in 2017 and ~64kg now.

Picture 31

I achieve this with the Stage 1 Biobloc appliance. I designed this in the late 1960s based on Schwartz's screw appliance. There have been many copies since but I think the Stage 1 Biobloc is still the best. Most hold on to the teeth or are screwed into the bone to reduce the force on the teeth and several of them push on the teeth with springs which is bound to cause root resorption. But the Stage one pushes very gently on the palate as well as the teeth to divide the force between them. After some research I discovered that the natural rate of tooth or bone movement was about 1/16th of a millimetre a day (less than a hairsbreadth) but most other expansion appliances are moved faster or slower or at different intervals.

I wrote a paper in 1977 describing this which was applauded by Professor Robert Moyers, the top orthodontist of the time but it was ignored by almost everyone else. Many clinicians also expand the lower jaw to match the upper, but the mandible is a single bone and cannot widen, so the teeth have to tilt which can damage them. I do not expand the lower jaw but use "shelves" on the upper appliance so the lowers can widen themselves over time, as a result of natural tongue posture. The shelves also encourage the mandible to slide forward.

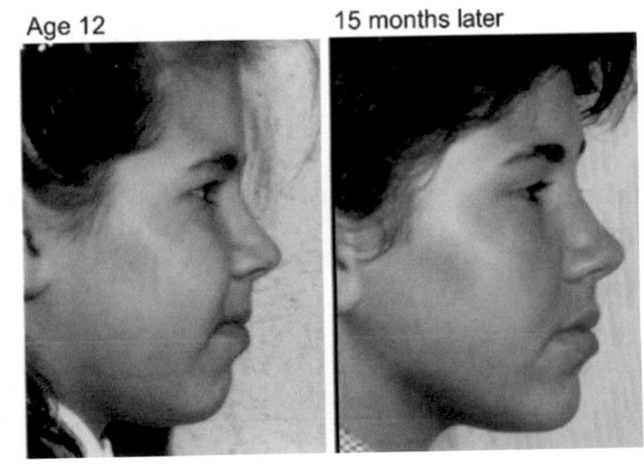

Picture 35

Subsequently (1983) I showed that the Stage 1 expansion was very stable, but that article too was ignored. I always seemed to be doing the "Wrong" thing at the "Wrong" time. In the 1980s some of my patient's parents started to comment on the improvement in facial appearance which I am ashamed to say I had hardly noticed (see picture 35).

At that time and even now, most orthodontists believed there was little that can be done to change the appearance and so they carried on aligning the teeth which is what they were taught. However it seemed to me that many patients were more concerned with their appearance than the straightness of the teeth.

I wanted to know if treatment really made a difference to the face. So I collected a series of identical twins and treated one myself and sent the other to an orthodontist. It is not easy to persuade parents to allow their children to be experimented on and it took several years to collect six pairs. When I compared them after treatment, I was really surprised.

I asked a panel of ten postgraduates to judge their appearance before and after treatment but without telling them how they had been treated (a blind study). Most of the twins treated by orthodontists were judged to be better looking before treatment, probably because I has asked the orthodontists which twin they wished to treat, however, after treatment everyone of them was judged to look worse. In contrast all but one of the Orthotropic cases looked better. This picture shows one of the pairs, note how Orthotropics pushed the "sicking out front teeth" further forward so the lower jaw could be taken even further forward. (see picture 36)

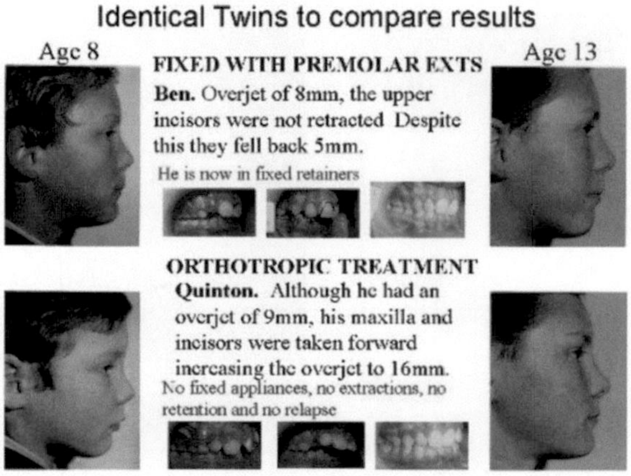

Identical Twins to compare results

Age 8

Age 13

FIXED WITH PREMOLAR EXTS

Ben. Overjet of 8mm, the upper incisors were not retracted Despite this they fell back 5mm.

He is now in fixed retainers

ORTHOTROPIC TREATMENT

Quinton. Although he had an overjet of 9mm, his maxilla and incisors were taken forward increasing the overjet to 16mm.

No fixed appliances, no extractions, no retention and no relapse

Picture 36

There was little difference in the straightness of the teeth immediately after treatment, but ten years later all those treated with fixed appliances had re-crowded to an unacceptable extent, except one who was wearing a permanent retainer. Again to my surprise, in all the Orthotropic cases, the teeth were still straight ten years after treatment. I think that was because we had improved their posture. I did other research which convinced me that Orthotropics, encouraged 10 or more millimetres of forward growth (Mew 2015), while fixed appliances restricted forward growth. I also compared excellent results treated by either Orthodontics or Orthotropics to find that the latter were considered Highly Significantly better looking. (Mew 2015). I also found that Orthotropics prevented almost all impacted canines (Mew & Mew.2015) but could only get them published in foreign Journals.

Almost all my British orthodontic colleagues think Orthotropics is nonsense, but when I talk to them I realise that they know little about it, or about posture generally and I don't think either are taught in British schools. Lots of clinicians in many different countries now do Orthotropics to varying standards. However the quality of the final result is highly dependent on how far they reduce the Indicator Line, and few British students are even taught what that is.

A lot depends on how far forward the upper incisors are taken forward. I would recommend that parents seeking treatment look carefully at the facial changes of a number of cases as that is a better indicator of quality than the alignment of the teeth. They might also ask their future Orthotropist how far they intend to reduce the Indicator Line.

The further forward the front teeth are taken, the better the face looks, but the longer the treatment takes and the more skill required, so the end result can vary widely. For instance the two brothers below both achieved room for all the teeth in a nice line but one has more forward growth and plenty of room for the tongue while the other is marginal and in my opinion will slowly relapse over time. (see pictures 37 and 38)

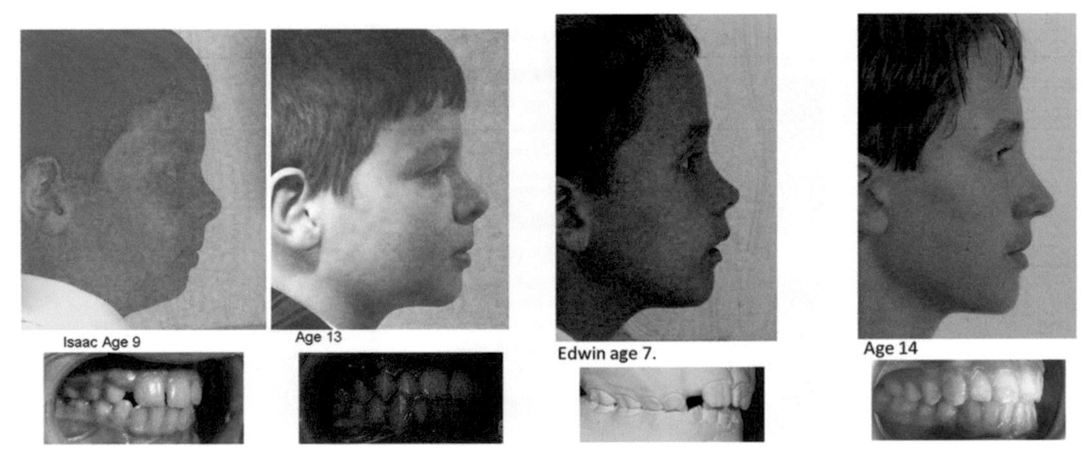

Picture 37 Picture 38

Recently there has been a revival of maxillary expansion although I used to be severely criticized for using it. Some of these new appliances are quite traumatic and I think their long-term stability is suspect but they can create some forward growth which improves the appearance of the face and avoids extractions. As a result it has again become popular but orthodontists have always had difficulty in bringing the lower jaw forward to match the upper.

Surgery. These days dentists tend to recommend surgery for any child or young adult whose lower jaw is back by more than four or five millimetres. This is because hundreds of research projects have shown that fixed orthodontic appliances cannot bring the lower jaw forward by more than two or perhaps three millimetres and it is now accepted that you can't make the mandible grow more than that. Orthodontists quote this research to ridicule my claims to make the jaw grow ten or even twenty millimetres, but of course I use different methods.

I initially trained as a jaw surgeon so know how traumatic this can be, the jaw is cut unto three sections and the middle one is then bolted together in a forward position. About 1000 British children and young adults have jaw surgery each year and the only alternative they are given is compromise treatment, just tilting the teeth so they meet and their parents are told "there is no other way". This is quite untrue.

This dismissal upset me so much that I collected 11 cases where children had come to me because they had been told they needed surgery. In most cases I had encouraged one or both jaws to grow forward ten or more millimetres with Orthotropics. I then sent these records to every member of the British General Dental Council (GDC). (see pictures 39 and 40)

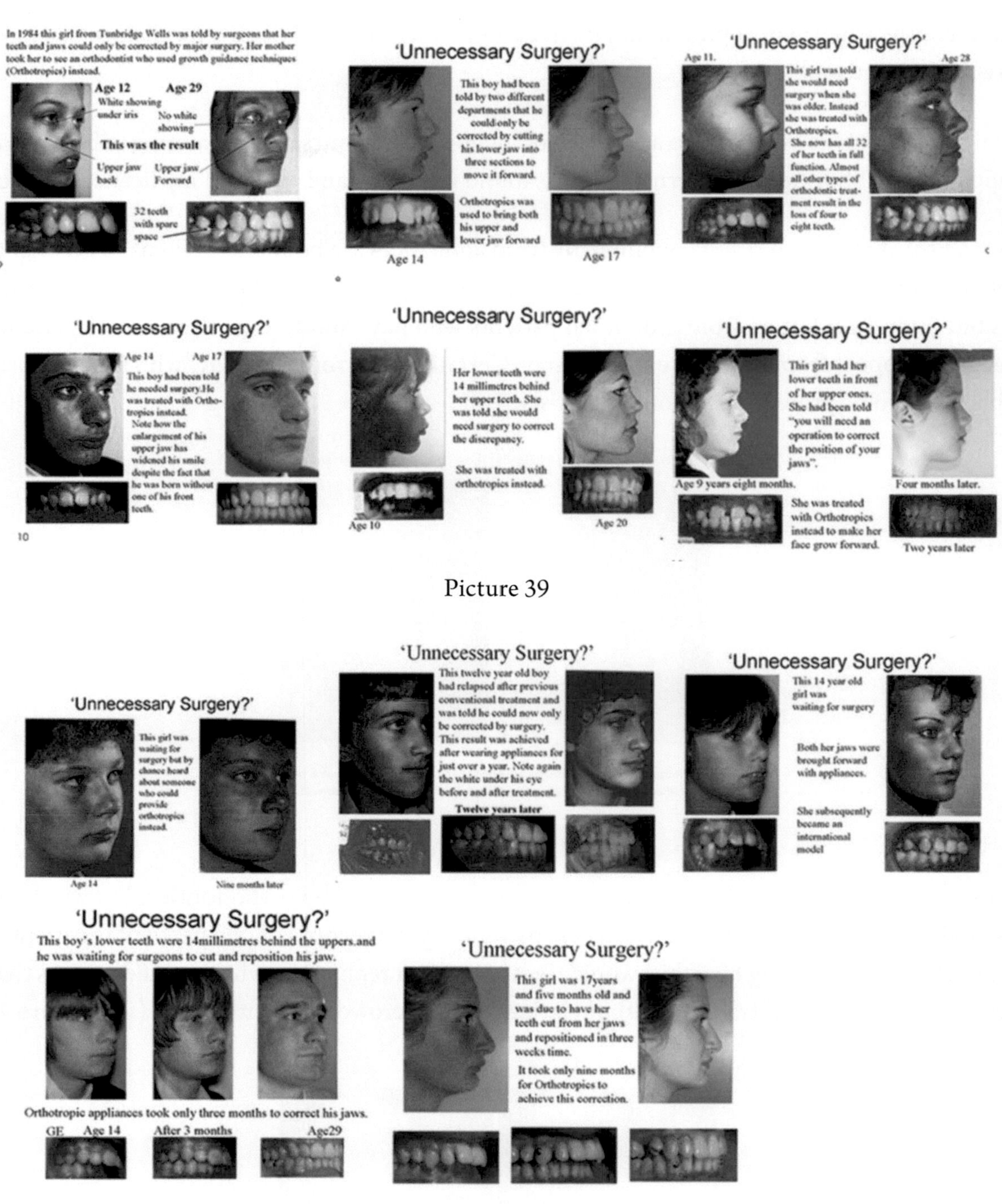

Picture 39

Picture 40

The GDC General committee agreed that the research should be considered by the Standards committee, but the Executive intervened to block this and the cases were never considered. Since then nearly 20,000 children and young adults have had surgery, much of which I am sure was unnecessary. I doubt if any of them were told there was a non-surgical alternative.

I wrote or lobbied all those I thought might be able to right this obvious wrong, over 50, MPs, Heads of departments, Government authorities, individuals and Colleagues. Most responded, many showed sympathy, but none were willing or able to change anything. The orthodontists, a large and powerful body, maintained

I had no evidence, when in my opinion they do not know either the cause or cure for malocclusion, yet alone how to achieve good looking faces.

The final response of the GDC was to accuse me of "deliberate dishonesty" for claiming to be able to change facial appearance. They held an internal enquiry, found me guilty and removed my licence to practice.

In general, I think the facial results obtained by fixed appliances are poor and it seems to me that the only faces orthodontists show are the surgical ones. It is not surprising that they do not disclose their facial failures but often I get letters from individual patients who have suffered (see picture 41), and who find they get little support from elsewhere in dentistry. Certainly not from the GDC who far from protecting the public seem to be protecting the orthodontists.

Mary. Age 12 and age 15 following three years HG and extractions.

Her father a medical doctor, complained to the British Dental Council but they rejected him because it was an acceptable standard of treatment.

Picture 41

It is not easy for the public to know how often faces are damaged by orthodontics. However there was one research project which explored its success by sending the records of one particular patient to every orthodontist in Briton, asking how they would treat him. Most replied but what amazed me was that nearly all of them recommended extractions although there was no crowding in either jaw. (see picture 42)

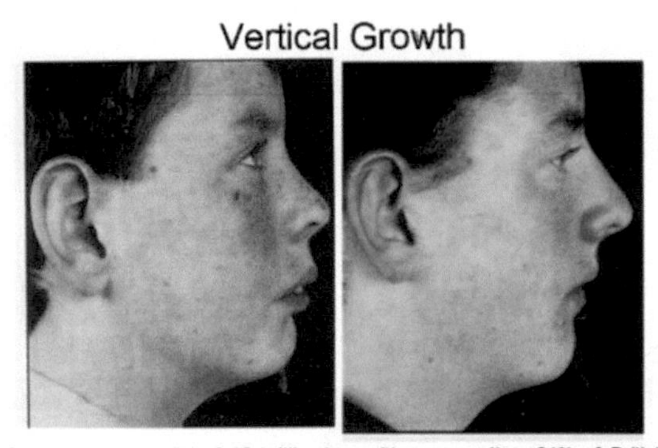

Brian had an overjet of 10 millimeters with no crowding. 91% of British orthodontists recommended treatment with first pre-molar extractions and 63% recommended retractive head gear. He was then treated with fixed appliances. Ten lay judges rated his facial appearance as 55 before treatment and 42 after. By kind permission of Dental Update.

Picture 42

His maxilla was quite far forward to start with and the paper is now 20 years old, but I suspect that the extraction ratio would still be around 80% despite there being no crowding. I think this is appalling.

The girl below shows how difficult it can be to assess facial appearance after orthodontic treatment because the head often tilts, bringing the chin forward (see picture 43). It is better to align the forehead than any other feature.

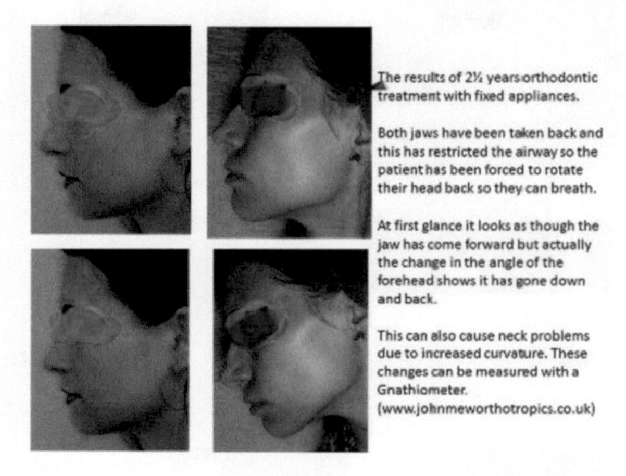

Picture 43

Forward Growth. Retruded faces may be normal in civilised populations, but they are not natural and go with crowded teeth, Jaw joint problems and sleepless nights. The time to achieve forward growth is before eight years old, but few children are treated this young.

If the jaws grow forward there will be more room for the wisdom teeth see picture, so they are less likely to be impacted. (see picture 44)

WHAT ACTUALLY HAPPENS?

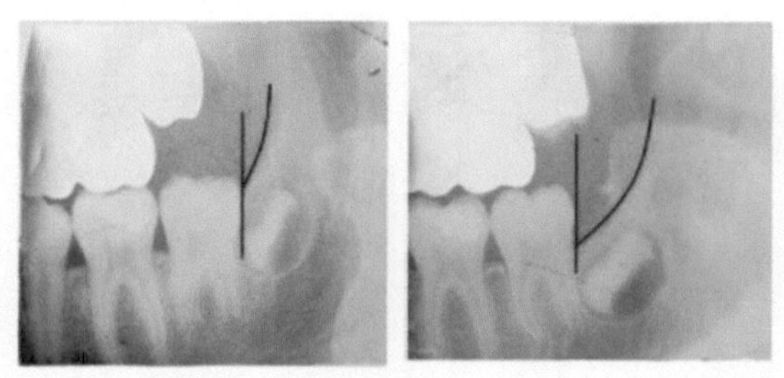

X-rays of Philip Age 14. **After nine 9 months orthotropics.**
Note that the assending ramus has moved back 7mm relative to the unerrupted wisdom which now has room to errupt.

Picture 44

Here are a few examples of faces that have been brought forward by Orthotropics. Note the double chins and flattened faces before treatment. (see pictures 45 to 67)

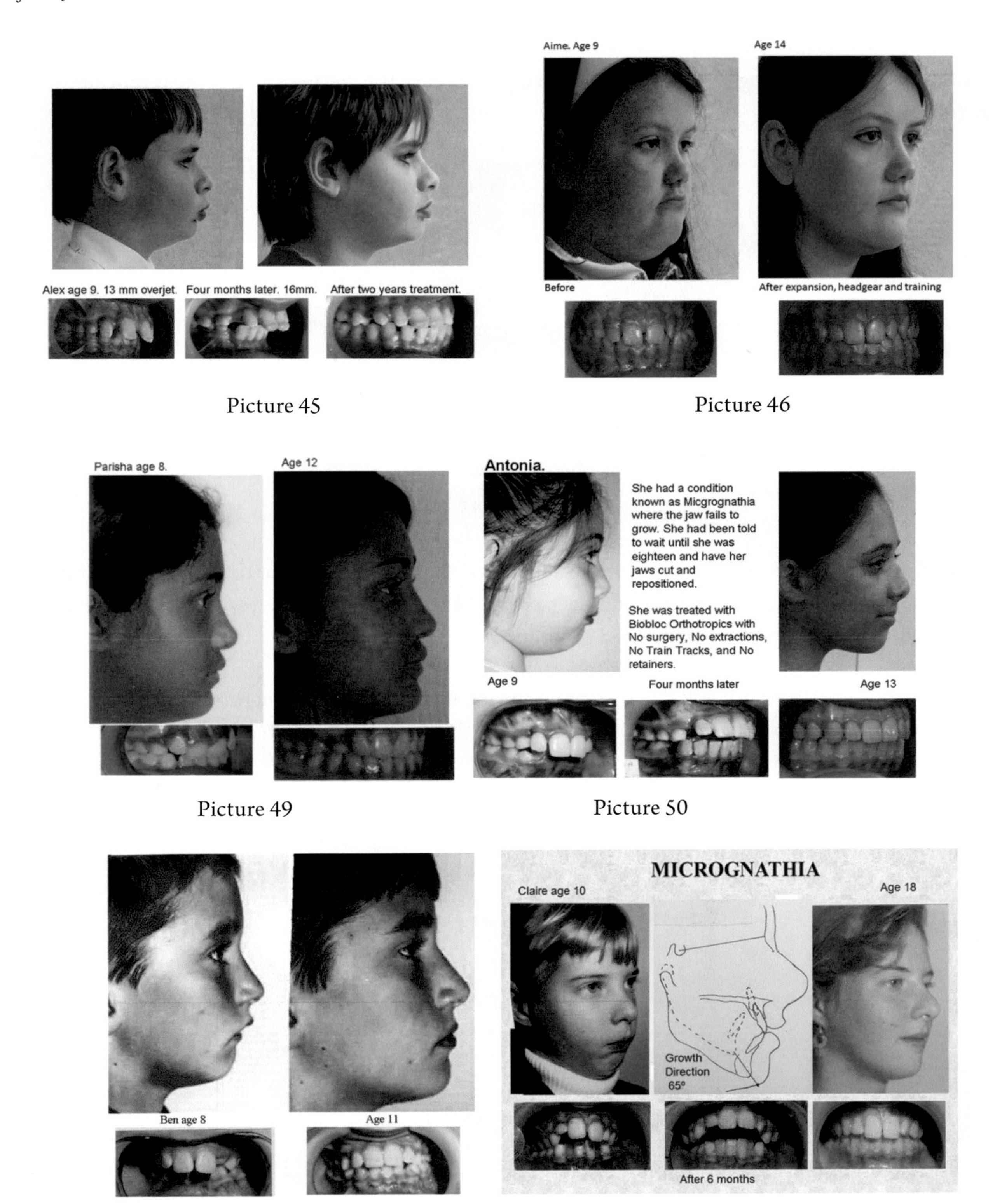

Picture 45

Picture 46

Picture 49

Picture 50

Picture 51

Picture 52

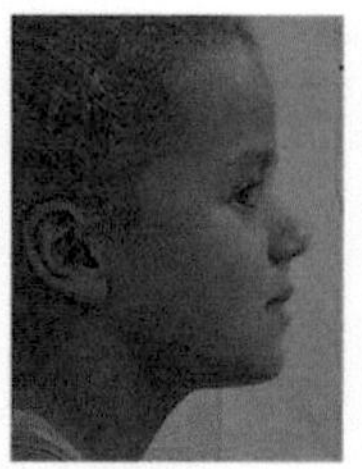

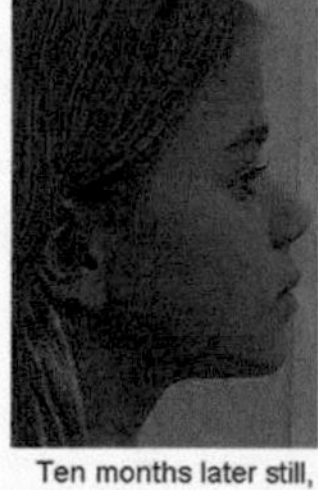

Kate Boswell age 8

Four months later, after Forward pull Head-gear and Stage 1

Ten months later still, after Stage 3

Picture 53

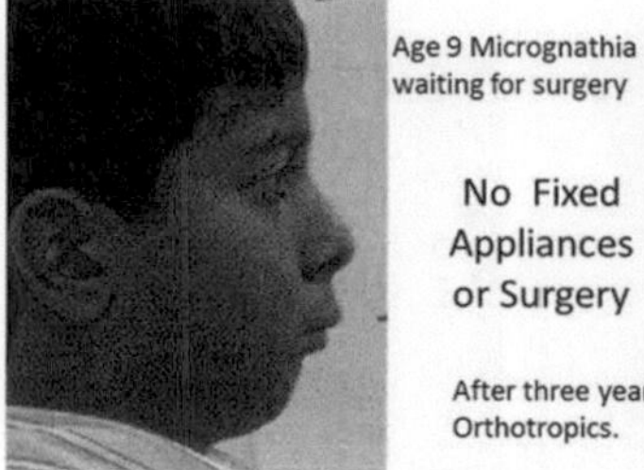

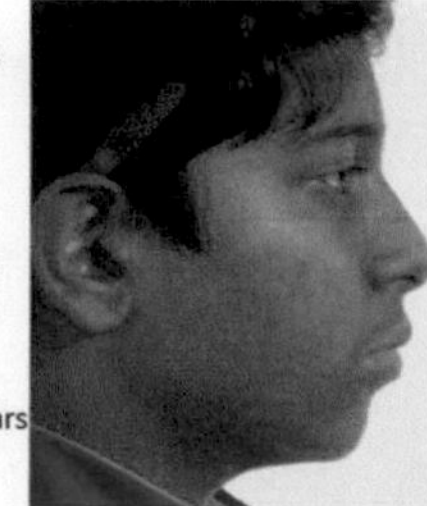

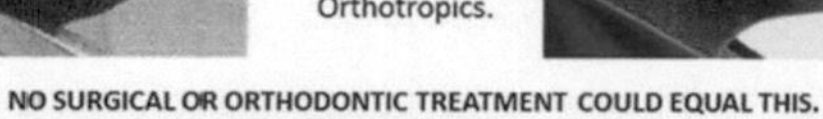

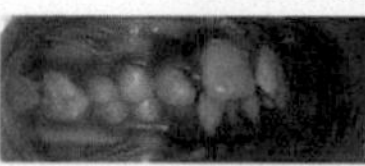

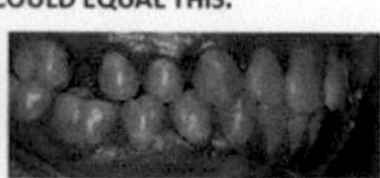

Both arches set back.

Jaws and Incisors moved forward.

Incisors have up righted in forward position.

Picture 54

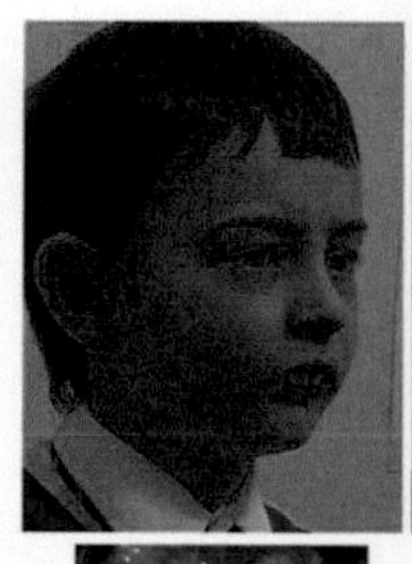

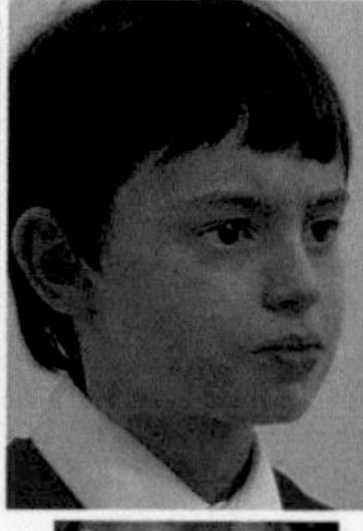

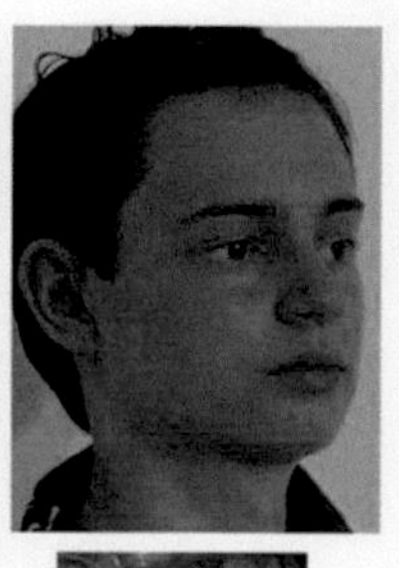

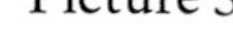

Robin age 9. "Micrognathia will need surgery".

14 months later. No surgery.

Five years later. Night wear only.

Picture 55

Jenny age 10y 7m.

Age 13y 3m

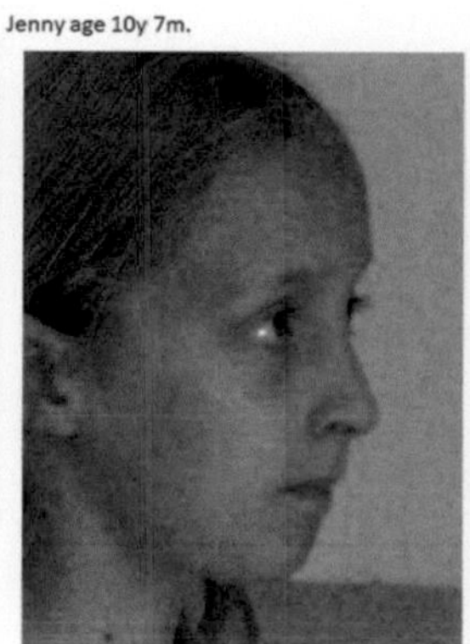

Before

After 2nd cycle.

Picture 56

Jamini Age 14

Age 15

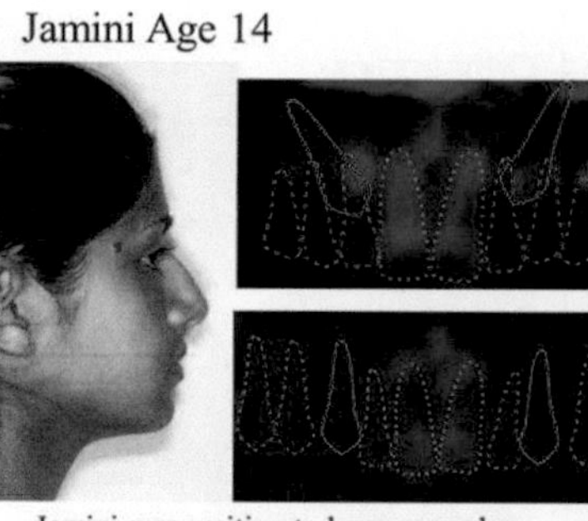

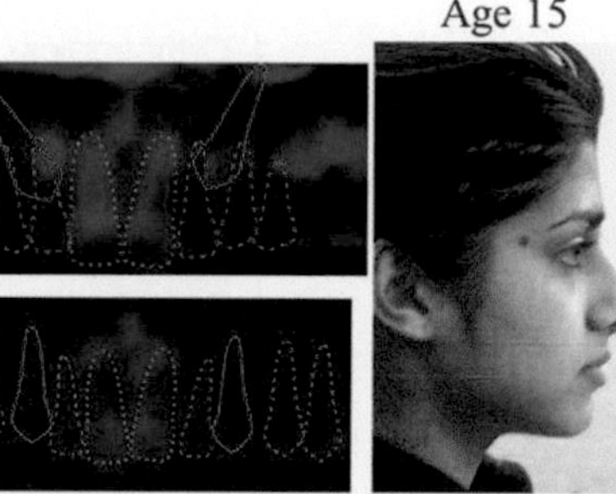

Jamini was waiting to have premolar extractions and surgery to expose her canines. Orthotropics advanced the maxilla and mandible providing room without extractions.

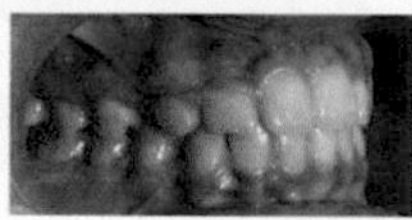

Picture 57

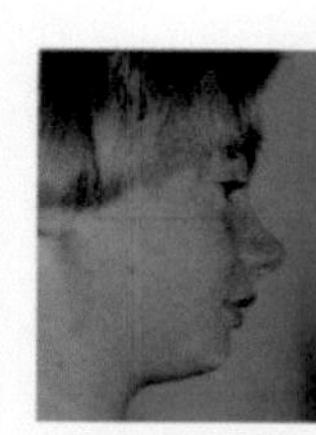

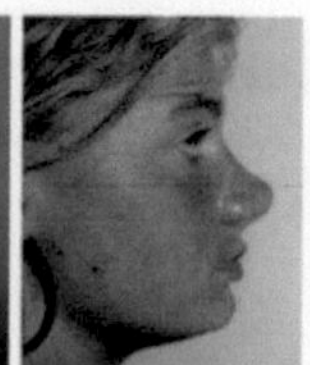

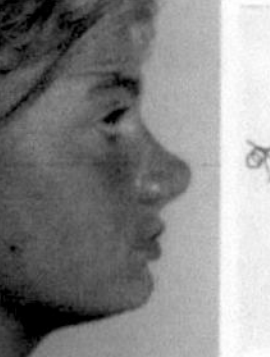

Lucy - Aged 12

Age 14

Age 12 & 14

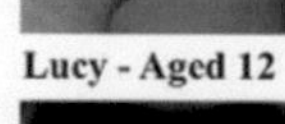

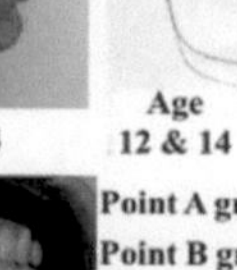

Point A grew 6mm
Point B grew 13mm
Growth direction 37 degre

Picture 58

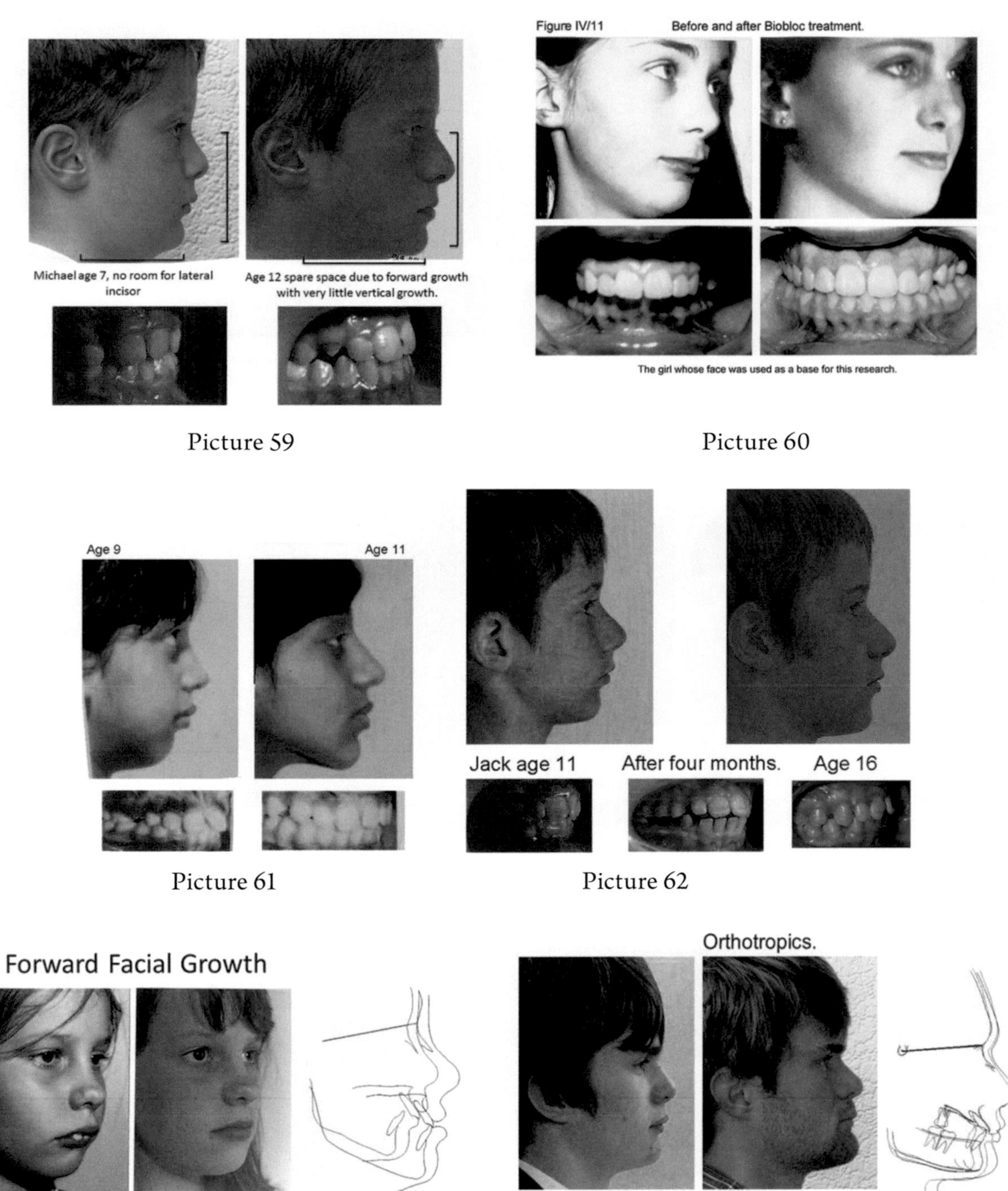

Picture 59

Picture 60

Picture 61

Picture 62

Picture 63

Picture 64

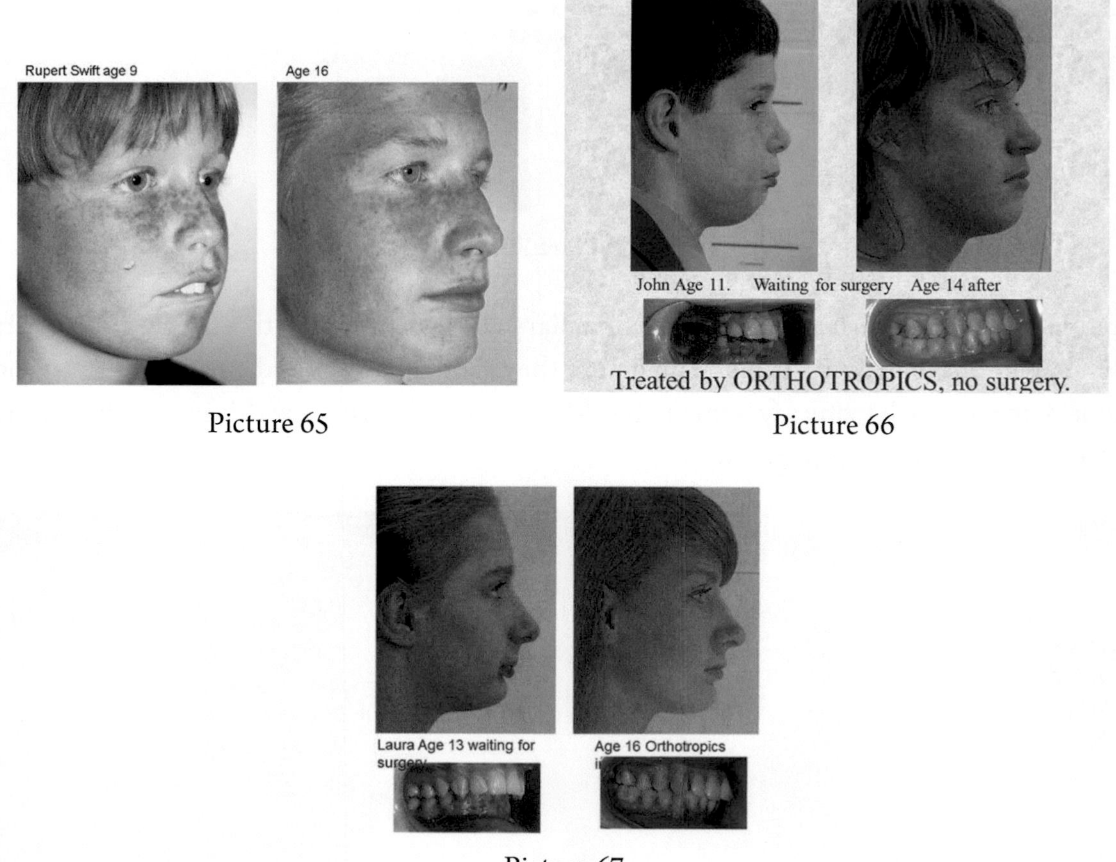

Picture 65

Picture 66

Picture 67

Older patients. While Orthotropic treatment is intended to be preventative, many patients need treatment older than eight. Several of the cases above were older than this and treatment is still possible in the twenties. (see pictures 68 and 69)

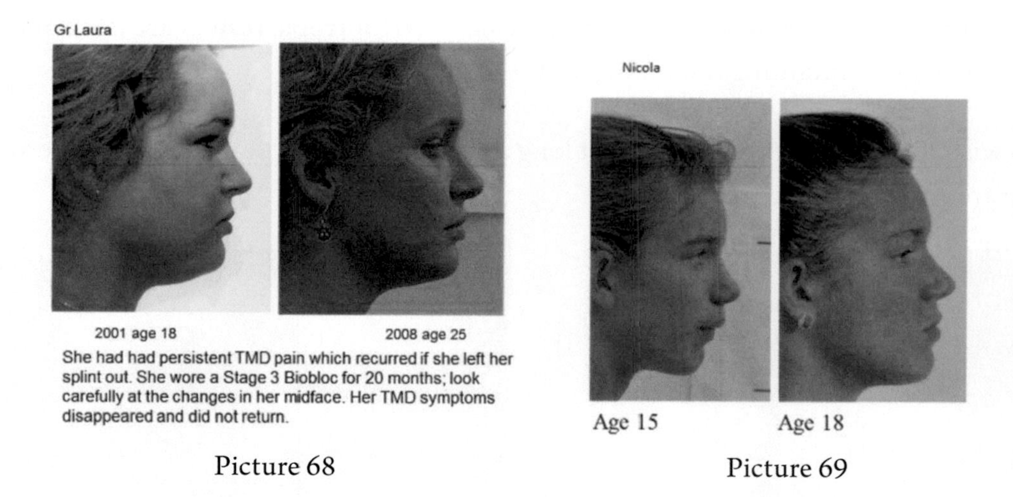

Picture 68

Picture 69

After twenty-five change becomes much slower but bones can still change shape at any age. This lady achieved a worthwhile change in her thirties. (see picture 70)

An adult aged 37 who had semi-rapid orthotropics.
Before treatment and 18 months later.

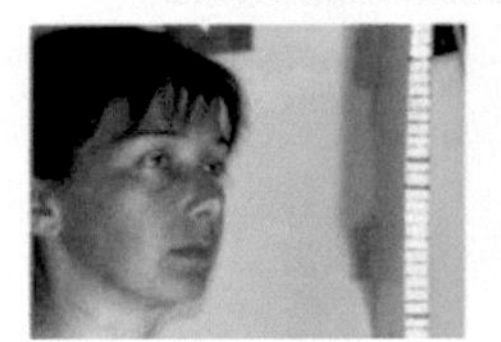
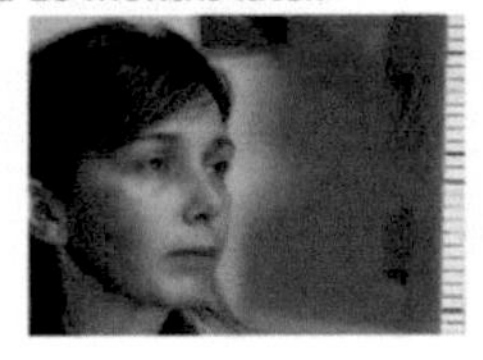

Picture 70

I am currently widening a 41 year old to his full maxillary width of 44mm with a Biobloc Stage 1. His teeth have tilted slightly but if he corrects his oral posture they should upright and currently there is no sign of gum or bone damage which many say is inevitable. Most of my colleagues say this impossible without some form of surgical intervention. (see picture 71)

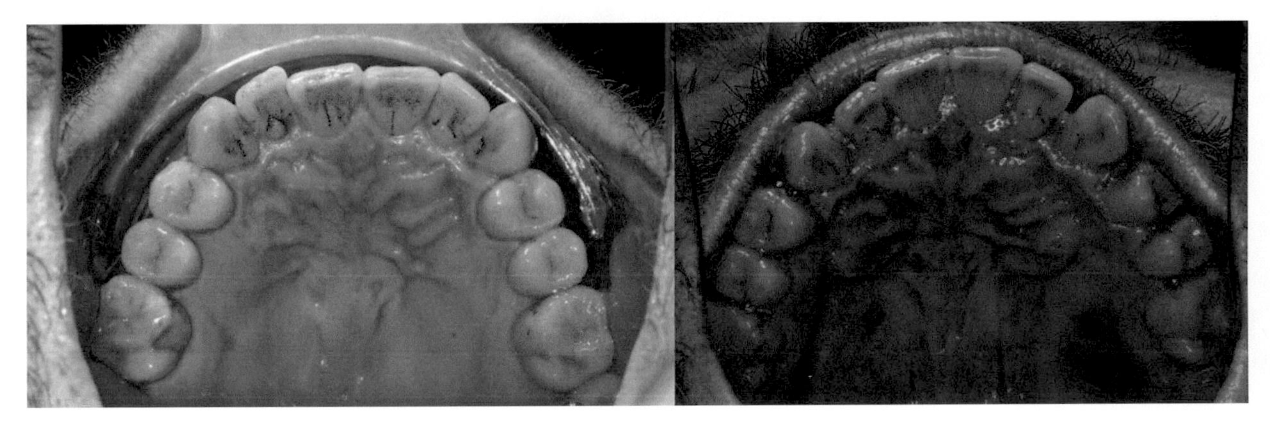

Picture 71

Stability. If teeth are moved mechanically with fixed appliances there is a strong tendency for them to relapse afterwards. Orthodontists avoid this by holding the teeth in position with fixed or removable retainers, this is effective, but they need to be worn indefinitely. Usually Orthotropic results are permanent but it does depend on the patient maintaining their oral posture. (see picture 36)

Few patients wish to return to the orthodontist long after treatment but sometimes I come across them by chance. Here are two. (see pictures 72 and 73)

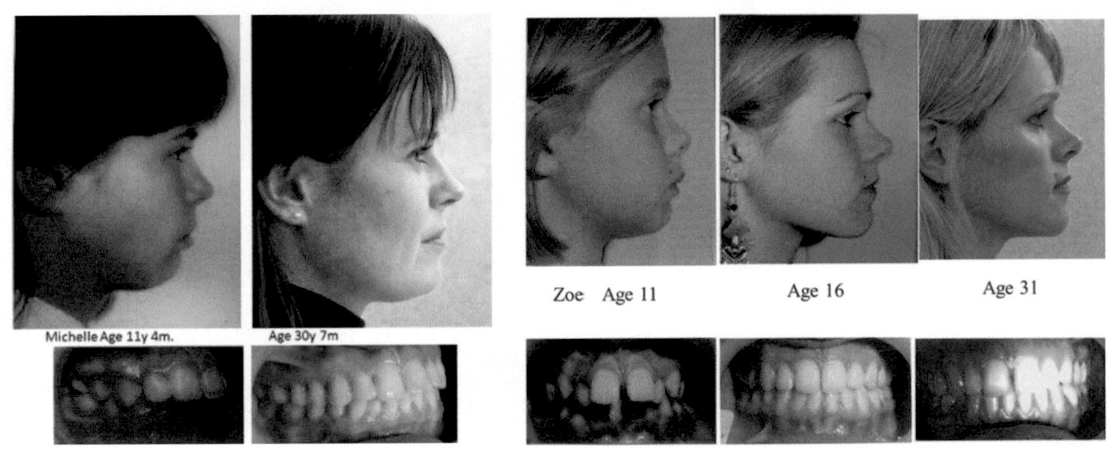

Picture 72

Picture 73

Alternative treatments. There are other methods of treatment for both older and younger patients.

Invisalign. This is a series of clear plastic aligners which fit over the teeth and hardly show. They are quite effective at aligning the teeth and I can see them displacing the fixed appliances about which I am so critical. However they also have some problems.

They can be designed to widen the arch, but in my experience, tend to retract the incisors and cause a downswing of the face in the process. I don't think they can yet move the whole dentition forward but they may overcome this one day. (see picture 74)

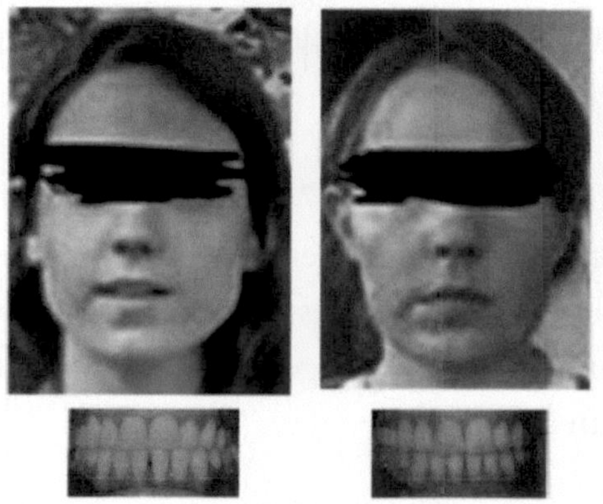

Postural and facial changes following a course of Invisalign.

Picture 74

Another possibly more severe problem is that the Invisalign appliances prop the bite open slightly and have difficulty controlling Roll, Pitch and Yaw. These are when the upper or lower jaw tilts sideways, back and forth or twists. If this happens it usually requires surgery to correct it. Let us hope they can learn to avoid this in future, otherwise youngsters who just wanted a small dental improvement have found themselves requiring major surgery.

Orthopaedic Appliances. These are sometimes called Functional Appliances, I was trained to use them at dental school and developed Orthotropics from them. They aim to alter the function and position of the maxilla and mandible. They are usually able to bring the upper and lower teeth into contact and will get a good result if the muscle tone is good, however they do not seem able to make the jaw grow and if the posture is poor Orthopaedic appliances may increase vertical growth considerably. Their problem is that they do not train the patients to keep their mouth closed.

Myobrace. This a preformed orthotropic appliance sold in different sizes and forms rather than being made individually. Naturally it is much less expensive but again does not train the patients to keep their mouth closed. Exercises are used to train the children to improve their posture but if they do not achieve this they are likely to be unsuccessful.

Advice on finding the right clinician. If young mothers follow the advice I have given their baby should have no problems. Most infants under six look appealing to everyone, this is an instinct planted within all of us to protect them, as in reality babies are demanding and very selfish. However after the age of 8 many of them may become quite plain (see the section in chapter 1 on the Indicator Line). The sad thing is that by the time this is noticed, much of the damage has been done.

The Indicator Line can recognise poor growth from under the age of four. so I would recommend all mothers to measure this. If it is high they will need advice from a clinician. Writing in 2022, few dentists or Orthodontists are trained in Growth Guidance (Orthotropics) especially in Britain and you may need to take this book with you for them to understand.

Older children will need active treatment to reverse any damage. Some clinicians claim to practice Orthotropics although they have not been trained and I would suggest that you take two essential measurements so that you can measure your child's needs and monitor any treatment. These are The Indicator Line and the Inter-Molar Width (the minimum distance between the upper first molar at gum level).

As I said the Indicator Line should measure about 27 millimetres at four and increase at 1mm per year until growth stops shortly after puberty. This is a very sensitive measurement and 3 millimetres can make the difference between a good looking and ordinary result. I do not have precise measurements for the Inter-Molar Width but it should be around 38mm by the age of ten and 42mm for a fully grown woman and 44mm for a man. The average British man is 33.5mm.

I would suggest that you discuss this with your clinician before any treatment and check the two measurements if you are concerned with progress. I should add that in older children with high Indicator Lines a full correction may not be possible. Here we are on a sliding scale, full correction should provide an excellent face with plenty of room for all 32 teeth, while higher Indicator Lines may result in impacted wisdom teeth or the extraction four or even eight teeth.

It is quite reasonable for a clinician to decide in advance to aim for a reasonable or excellent result depending on the final Indicator Line and the fee would vary depending on the time and skill involved. This of course should be a matter of discussion before treatment.

A final word. For those young mothers for whom I wrote this book. I hope you have found it helpful rather than frightening but the time to take action is at birth. Suckle your baby if you possibly can, and make sure baby takes a big mouthful of your breast and pumps on it. If you can manage this for 26 months delaying spoon or cup feeding until they are ready for it (baby led weening), then you have set them on the right road.

One day in the future I hope almost everyone will grow up with natural good looking faces, with no stuffy noses, blocked ears or jaw joint problems and live to a healthy age without sleep apnoea.

About the author.

Professor JOHN MEW. BDS. Lond, LDS RCS Eng. MFGDP (UK). M Orth Edin.

Born in 1928, his father was an orthodontist. John is a lateral thinker and dyslexic, who found exams difficult. After qualifying in 1953, he studied Maxilo-facial surgery at Queen Victoria Hospital East Grinstead, before moving to orthodontics in 1965. In the 1960s He created the first Dental Association Benevolent Raffle against considerable opposition, which subsequently raised approaching a million pounds. For many years he remained very much within the establishment becoming president of the Southern Counties Branch of the British Dental Association in 1971. He has been honoured with membership of the Faculty of General Dental Practitioners, life membership of the British Dental Association, and Fellowship of the International College of Dentists. In 2010 he was honoured with "outstanding achievement awards" both by the International Association of Orthodontists and by the International Functional Association

His surgical training, gave him the opportunity to study occlusal and Temporo Mandibular Joint problems. He later developed an interest in facial changes during both natural growth and orthodontic treatment. This led him to explore the cause and cure of facial deformities.

In 1958 he put forward the 'Tropic Premise' "The aetiology of malocclusion: can the Tropic Premise assist our understanding". British Dental Journal. 1981:**151;** :296-302. which suggested that malocclusion was a 'Postural Deformity' and that irregular teeth were not necessarily inherited. He became concerned that the mechanics of orthodontic treatment could be harmful to facial growth, and over the subsequent 20 years developed the concept of facial 'Growth Guidance' [Orthotropics] and the 'Biobloc' system of treatment. At the time the establishment labelled him a maverick and applied considerable political, legal and financial pressure to prevent him from using many procedures that are now commonplace.

He has written a large number of scientific papers and three full length text books about his technique "Biobloc", the second of which is now in its 4th edition and has been translated into seven different languages. He has also lectured and/or taught in most countries in the world, where he has set up many study groups. In 2021 he put forward the Mastantlos Hypothesis to explain the widespread development of facial dysmorphia.

Sports. Always a keen competitor, he played rugby football until he was 50. At the age of 18 he learnt to fly a Tiger Moth, and subsequently took up fixed wing gliding and later hang gliding, making an attempt on the British Endurance Record which was frustrated by the weather. At the age of 22 he designed and built his own sports car, fabricating much of it from scratch, and winning the first speed event he entered it for. From 1957 to 1968 he took up motor racing seriously, moving from formula three to formula one, and was one of the last successful private entrants in the sport, entering events all over Europe. In 1963 he twice broke the Formula One club circuit record at Brands Hatch, beating times set by World Champions Jim Clarke, and John Surtees.

A keen sailor. In 1958 he was selected for the British Team for the first post-war challenge for the Americas Cup, unfortunately due to subsequent changes he did not take part in the event itself. In 1971 he was selected to crew John Prentice the captain for the British 'International Fourteen' dingy racing team in Annapolis,

USA where Britain came second. In 1974 John in his International 14 'Achilles' with his crew Michael Moss took second place in the World Championship anniversary race at Cowes UK.

Other Interests. A philosopher at heart with an interest in human sciences he has just completed a book on social anthropology. More pragmatically he is interested in the construction and repair of ancient buildings and in 1999 he built a reproduction castle on an island in a lake. This captured the public imagination and received several national awards including the "Best New Home in Britain". The nephew of a successful inventor, he himself has many inventions (successful and unsuccessful) to his credit. In the past he has also been a garage proprietor, jousted in medieval armour, and at the age of 70 bungee jumped in Australia.

Home. Widowed in 2013 from his wife of 50 years with three children, he is especially interested in the construction and repair of ancient buildings. He lives in his castle on an island in a lake in East Sussex (South of London).

Printed in the United States
by Baker & Taylor Publisher Services

Printed in the United States
by Baker & Taylor Publisher Services